Managing Personality Disordered Offenders

Managing Personality Disordered Offenders
A Pathways Approach

Edited by

Colin Campbell
Consultant Forensic Psychiatrist
South London and Maudsley NHS Foundation Trust and
King's College London, UK

Jackie Craissati
Consultant Forensic and Clinical Psychologist
Psychological Approaches CIC, London, UK

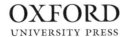

OXFORD
UNIVERSITY PRESS

OXFORD
UNIVERSITY PRESS

Great Clarendon Street, Oxford, OX2 6DP,
United Kingdom

Oxford University Press is a department of the University of Oxford.
It furthers the University's objective of excellence in research, scholarship,
and education by publishing worldwide. Oxford is a registered trade mark of
Oxford University Press in the UK and in certain other countries

Published in the United States of America by Oxford University Press
198 Madison Avenue, New York, NY 10016, United States of America

British Library Cataloguing in Publication Data

Data available

Library of Congress Control Number: 2018931002

ISBN 978–0–19–879187–4

Printed in Great Britain by
Ashford Colour Press Ltd, Gosport, Hampshire

Foreword

In my review of people with mental health problems and learning disabilities in the criminal justice system in 2009, the high prevalence of personality disorder in prison populations was striking, as was the large proportion of mental health in-reach team caseloads taken up with personality disorder. Despite this, there was no formal provision of services for people with personality disorder in prison.

In my report, I suggested that the development of personality disorder-specific services would play a significant role in improving prison mental health services and achieving 'equivalence of services' for offenders with personality disorder. One of the key recommendations of the report was that the Department of Health, the (then) National Offender Management Service, and the National Health Service should develop an interdepartmental strategy for the management of all levels of personality disorder within both the health service and the criminal justice system. Further, I recommended that this strategy should cover the management of offenders with personality disorder into and through custody, and also their management in the community.

Following public consultation, the response from the UK government in 2011 was the joint commissioning—by the Department of Health and the National Offender Management Service—of the Offender Personality Disorder pathway, a new approach to the management of individuals whose offending behaviour was likely to be linked to personality disorder. I was delighted to see that the underlying principles of the Offender Personality Disorder pathway were innovative and, as recommended in my report, focused on the provision of a pathway of services from community to community, which is jointly led and delivered by health and criminal justice staff.

This book, looking at the London Pathways Partnership, a consortium of mental health trusts, describes how they implemented the Offender Personality Disorder pathway, in partnership with prison and probation services, in London and the surrounding area. The book strikes a balance between a scholarly review of the relevant evidence bases, including those from services outside of the UK, and providing a practical guide to their approach to developing and delivering services in a range of secure and community settings. The authors, all of whom have extensive experience of developing and delivering services for offenders with personality disorder, describe what has worked well, and are transparent in highlighting the mistakes they made and the obstacles they encountered. Covering a diverse range of topics, from training to case formulation and service-user involvement to commissioning, they make some thought-provoking proposals for how these services might develop over the next years.

This book will be an invaluable resource for the growing workforce in the Offender Personality Disorder pathway and for health and criminal justice professionals whose work inevitably brings them into contact with this complex group of offenders. It offers new ways of thinking about service development and innovative solutions to challenging problems.

The Rt Hon. The Lord Bradley,
House of Lords,
London.

Bradley KJ. The Bradley Report: Lord Bradley's review of people with mental health problems and learning disabilities in the criminal justice system. London: Department of Health; 2009.

Foreword

There is little doubt that if we are to provide effective treatment for the many individuals within criminal justice systems inflicted with personality disorder, we will need to be innovative and think well outside the box. Not only are these disorders prevalent, but also they involve a level of complexity and a diversity of problems that challenge conventional approaches. What is needed is a comprehensive systemic approach that reflects the complex needs of personality disordered offenders. The framework presented in this volume nicely fits the bill. Rather than taking current treatment models and considering how they could best be delivered within the criminal justice system, the authors take the broader and more challenging route of developing an overall pathway of care that encapsulates current evidence-based thinking about what works and what is needed for comprehensive care. Although the model incorporates elements that reflect the context of its development, it rests on principles that have wider currency and there is much that is appealing to the pathway proposed.

The overall approach is very much in line with the findings of current outcome studies. If we know anything about treating personality disorder, it is that good outcomes depend on structured and consistent care. Structure in this sense is not simply a matter of how treatment is organized and delivered but also incorporates the systemic and administrative contexts of care. Within such a system, change is brought about not only by the various interventions used across the pathway but also by the overall system continuously providing corrective experiences that progressively challenge and change core aspects of the disorder.

The pathway proposed wisely recognizes that an effective system requires a single philosophy of care shared by all involved. This is necessary if the different components of the pathway and different staff who are often engaged in very different activities are to work together in a seamless way. However, given the modest state of current knowledge, developing a common conception of the disorder presents something of a challenge. The authors propose a two-component framework consisting of attachment theory and the desistence model. While there seems little doubt that these are necessary ingredients of any comprehensive approach to care, time will tell whether they are also sufficient. Given the aetiological, developmental, and psychopathological complexity of personality disorder, something more comprehensive may ultimately be needed. However, the overall approach with its emphasis on conceptual and organizational clarity and an integrative evidence-based approach to care provides the kind of framework needed to treat personality disorder not only in criminal justice settings but also in healthcare systems. It is also the kind of structure that can readily grow and develop as our ideas about this disorder and its management evolve.

John Livesley
Professor Emeritus
Department of Psychiatry
University of British Columbia
Vancouver, BC, Canada

Preface

Personality disorder is undoubtedly a controversial topic, partly on account of the diagnostic problems that it poses, but more importantly its implications for the individual in terms of negative connotations and stigma. The picture is particularly complex in relation to those who have committed offences because of the well evidenced link between personality disorder and heightened risk of harm to others.

In our view, the offender personality disorder (OPD) pathway in the UK represents a truly original approach to tackling a complex and widespread concern; it achieves this with relatively few resources, adopting something of a public health approach rather than an illness management approach, with its systemic focus and its 'bottom-up' implementation. At the core of the OPD pathway lies a partnership approach – mental health and criminal justice services working together from commissioning to delivery. Partnership is, we would contest, a rather over used word, and in reality, rarely associated with transformative innovation. However, in the case of the OPD pathway, it really has represented a new way of doing things that has resolved many of the 'mad-bad' splits that fragment services for personality disordered offenders.

The London Pathways Partnership (LPP) adopted a consortium model to bring together the four London mental health trusts whose clinical leaders comprise the authors of this edited volume; this innovative partnership provided an exciting catalyst for the implementation of the OPD pathway innovations. In coming together to write this book, we wanted to show that collaboration can transcend traditional organizational boundaries, even in a resource-constrained competitive economy. The LPP has flourished after four years of immersion in the pathway: selfishly, writing this book has enabled us to pause and take stock, with a more objective eye. It has helped us to clarify in our own minds what has worked and where we need to be heading in the next few years.

We would like to take the opportunity to thank all of our LPP colleagues, whose hard work, enthusiasm, creativity and commitment have been central to the success of these services to date. We would also like to express our gratitude to our criminal justice and third sector partners, with particular thanks to Angus Cameron, Nick Joseph and Rachel O'Rourke.

Colin Campbell
Jackie Craissati
London
August 2018

Contents

Contributors

Pamela Attwell
Consultant Clinical Psychologist, Oxleas NHS Foundation Trust, London, UK

Mick Burns
Co-Commissioner PD Offender Pathway, NHS England, UK

Colin Campbell
Consultant Forensic Psychiatrist, South London and Maudsley NHS Foundation Trust and King's College London, UK

Jackie Craissati MBE
Consultant Forensic and Clinical Psychologist, Psychological Approaches CIC, London, UK

Rob Halsey
Consultant Forensic and Clinical Psychologist, Barnet, Enfield and Haringey Mental Health Trust, London, UK

Nikki Jeffcote
Consultant Clinical Psychologist, Oxleas NHS Foundation Trust, London, UK

Phil Minoudis
Consultant Clinical Psychologist, East London NHS Foundation Trust, London, UK

Emma Nicklin
Therapy and Service Development Lead, Barnet, Enfield and Haringey Mental Health Trust, London, UK

Chantal Scaillet
Clinical Psychologist, Oxleas NHS Foundation Trust, London, UK

Jake Shaw
Consultant Forensic Psychologist, Barnet, Enfield and Haringey Mental Health Trust, London, UK

Celia Taylor
Consultant Forensic Psychiatrist, East London NHS Foundation Trust, UK

Karen Van Gerko
Clinical Psychologist, Oxleas NHS Foundation Trust, London, UK

Chapter 1

Introduction

Colin Campbell and Jackie Craissati

The UK government's Offender Personality Disorder (OPD) strategy is one of the most significant developments in mental health and criminal justice services in recent years. Since its implementation in April 2012, the strategy has provided 236 new prison treatment places and 700 new places with psychologically informed management in prisons and in probation hostels. The entire probation caseload across custody and the community has been screened against criteria for inclusion in the pathway and services have been introduced in all probation areas to identify, assess, and jointly case manage offenders who meet the criteria.

At the same time, a workforce development programme has been put in place, directly linked to new service provision in prisons and the community, together with broader awareness-level training for mental health and criminal justice staff. An independent national evaluation of the entire OPD pathway has also been commissioned.

All of this has taken place in the context of unprecedented reorganization in the National Probation Service (NPS) and prison service and widespread cuts in public sector funding.

Despite the investment of £64 million and government backing, these services, as is the case with most services for personality disordered offenders, remain controversial. This is in part attributable to the controversial nature of personality disorder as a diagnosis, and the historical diffusion of responsibility for individuals with personality disorder when it is associated with antisocial behaviour between mental health and criminal justice services. Societal ambivalence about what to do with offenders with personality disorders complicates the picture further, particularly in relation to questions of criminal responsibility, risk, and rehabilitation. This is by no means only a UK problem, and the diversity of international approaches to the management of these individuals reflects both a recognition of the need to address the problem and the embryonic state of the relevant evidence bases.

The politics of personality disorder

The diagnosis of personality disorder continues to be controversial amongst service users, mental health professionals, academics, and the wider public.

Service user perspective

Critics of the diagnosis view it as the medicalization of distress or of extremes of normal behaviour, which necessarily involves a subjective judgement about 'normal behaviour'. While some find the diagnosis helpful in making sense of their experience, others find it stigmatizing and invalidating. It can be experienced as a criticism of who someone is, rather than what difficulties they may have, and can be used to exclude service users from accessing services.

Professional perspective

Some of these difficulties are reflected in the ongoing academic debate around the classification of these disorders [1]. Using current diagnostic criteria, most individuals meet criteria for more than one personality disorder and there is marked heterogeneity within any one diagnosis. That is, current criteria do not tend to neatly capture any one individual's difficulties in one diagnosis and those meeting the criteria for the same diagnosis may experience very different sets of difficulties from each other. Significantly, one of the most common diagnoses is Personality Disorder Unspecified or Not Otherwise Specified (NOS), where an individual does not meet the criteria for any one specific disorder [2]. The current classification systems also fail to acknowledge the increasing body of evidence indicating that personality disorder symptoms vary with time, independently of each other, and that, if they resolve, they tend not to recur [3]. Antisocial personality disorder, in particular, has long been subject to criticism due to its heavy reliance on behavioural criteria and failure to take into account social and contextual factors such as socioeconomic deprivation.

Societal perspective

However, the status of the diagnosis is not simply an academic point, as it informs views on the appropriateness of intervention in personality disorder and, if appropriate, who should provide it. If personality disorder represents extremes of normal behaviour, then do mental health services have any legitimate role in managing it? And if the extreme behaviour happens to be criminal behaviour, shouldn't it rightly be the domain of the criminal justice system? The status of the diagnosis also raises questions in relation to moral and criminal responsibility, together with societal expectations regarding the appropriateness of punishment and rehabilitation. Juries and judges are often most persuaded by a narrative that 'makes sense' and that is consistent with folk psychology. An offence committed by someone in response to command auditory hallucinations may make more sense to a jury, or may have a more convincing narrative, than one committed in the context of emotional dysregulation, where the accused may simply be seen as a criminal who lost their temper. Even mental health professionals tend to believe that individuals with personality disorder have more control over their behaviour and are, therefore, more responsible for their aggressive and violent behaviour [4]. Paradoxically, given the significant progress made in recent years in developing an evidence base for treatment of personality disorder, the relative lack of an evidence base in comparison to, say, depression, also informs societal views regarding the appropriateness, and likely effectiveness, of rehabilitation of offenders with a personality disorder.

Some of the legal and political implications of a personality disorder diagnosis are illustrated well by the case of the Norwegian, Anders Breivik. In July 2011, Breivik detonated a van bomb in the government district of Oslo, killing eight people, before shooting dead 69 participants of a Workers' Youth League summer camp on the island of Utøya. Prior to his trial, two court-appointed forensic psychiatrists diagnosed Breivik with paranoid schizophrenia [5]. This provoked considerable public outrage, as the legal insanity test in Norway simply requires the accused to have acted under the influence of psychosis at the time of the crime. This meant that Breivik could be found 'not legally accountable' and sentenced to compulsory treatment. Many felt cheated of the opportunity to punish Breivik and were worried that he might be freed too early. Following intense media coverage and public pressure, where those who undertook the initial evaluation were accused of incompetence, bias, and paranoia, a second psychiatric evaluation was undertaken, which concluded that Breivik was not psychotic but had severe narcissistic personality disorder and pseudologica fantastica (or pathological lying). This, too, resulted in public outcry, as many were frustrated that this diagnosis may result in a finite prison sentence, rather than indefinite detention, albeit in a psychiatric hospital. This is because the Norwegian criminal code has a maximum prison sentence of twenty-one years, with no additions for multiple victims. However, in particularly serious cases, the offender can be sentenced to additional protective detention.

Interestingly, Breivik himself did not want to be found 'not legally account-able', stating that he would prefer the death penalty to compulsory treatment [6]. He did not want to evade responsibility or avoid a trial. Indeed, he com-mitted his offences with the intent of achieving a high-profile trial.

What seems clear is that the basis for the public appetite for a diagnosis of per-sonality disorder is not straightforward. It may simply derive from a need to en-sure that the correct diagnosis is made to inform effective treatment. However, at times, it seems that the need for diagnosis is driven by a desire to ensure that the associated implications in relation to perceived responsibility, punishment, and removal from society follow from it.

All these issues contribute to societal ambivalence about whether or not per-sonality disordered offenders are deserving of treatment and rehabilitation, particularly given perhaps more obviously deserving causes in mental health and health more broadly.

What have other countries done?

Unsurprisingly, the question of how best to manage high-risk personality dis-ordered offenders is a global one. What is perhaps more striking is the breadth of responses to this question, which range from nothing whatsoever to well-established, complex services supported by specific legal frameworks.

Perhaps the best example of the latter type of response is the Dutch Ter Beschikking Stelling (TBS) system [7]. This is a provision within the Dutch penal code (literally meaning 'at the discretion of the state') for offenders who have committed serious violent or sexual offences, but who are assessed as being only partially responsible for their offences due to a mental disorder. Under the TBS system, offenders can be sentenced to an appropriate prison sentence, informed by the crime and assessed degree of responsibility, fol-lowed by an additional TBS order. This contrasts with the dichotomous ap-proach in the UK, where responsibility is diminished or is not, and there are five levels of responsibility ranging from fully responsible to not responsible (unfit to plead), where the offence is believed to have been caused entirely by the individual's mental disorder. As the prison sentence is imposed for the part of the offence for which the individual is deemed responsible, this decreases with each level of responsibility, from fully responsible to unfit to plead.

The purpose of the TBS order is to both protect society and provide treat-ment to reduce risk. The order is imposed for two years in the first instance but can be extended for as long as the court determines it is necessary in order to manage risk. The order is reviewed every two years by the court, which is also responsible for extending the order or discharging patients from it. Treatability and motivation to engage are not issues, as the primary aim of the TBS order is public protection and, if possible, rehabilitation. Offenders spend the first part of their order in a secure institution and, following successful unescorted leave, may be conditionally discharged by the court on the advice of the clinical team. If there are no incidents while under monitoring and supervision in the community, the TBS order is automatically unconditionally discharged after three years.

In addition to psychological treatment, the treatment model in TBS services places emphasis on therapeutic community principles, paid employment, relational security, and medication, particularly for sex offenders. The TBS system covers the entire pathway from high security to the community and includes long-stay facilities for those offenders who do not show any progress and do not reduce their risk, where the focus is on quality of life, rather than intensive treatment.

The TBS system has often been cited as one of the primary influences on the development of services for high-risk personality disordered offenders in the UK. However, some have argued that several key components were not adopted, particularly the legislative framework, and this has undermined the success of programmes in the UK. Another prominent influence on UK services has been the Violence Reduction Programme, developed and delivered in Saskatoon, Canada [8]. This programme is based on cognitive behavioural principles and social learning theory, and progress on identified treatment targets is assessed using standardized measures. In Saskatoon, the programme is delivered in the Regional Psychiatric Centre, a specialized unit within the Canadian Correctional System. Serving prisoners can volunteer to transfer to the service and can be returned to ordinary prisons if they do not progress or if they are involved in a violent incident.

In other jurisdictions, legislation allows for the civil commitment of offenders who continue to pose a high risk to others as the result of mental disorder following completion of a custodial sentence. The definition of a mental disorder is often broadly defined to include mental abnormality and personality disorder, such as in the Sexually Violent Predator legislation in the US (see Chapter 5).

Variation in how to manage high-risk personality disorder offenders is evident even within UK jurisdictions. In contrast to England and Wales, in Scotland and Northern Ireland there is no provision within mental health legislation for detention on the basis of a diagnosis of personality disorder alone. High-risk personality disorder offenders can only be detained within the criminal justice system and, therefore, only if they have been charged with, or convicted of, an offence [9].

Dangerous and Severe Personality Disorder programme

Although services for high-risk personality disordered offenders have existed in the UK for decades, most notably the democratic therapeutic community provision within the prison system, the most comprehensive attempt to address the needs of this population was the development of the Dangerous and Severe Personality Disorder (DSPD) programme. The catalyst for the development of this programme in England and Wales is often cited as the case of Michael Stone, who was convicted of the murder of Lin Russell and her daughter Megan and the attempted murder of Megan's sister Josie in 1996. An independent inquiry following his conviction found that Stone had a long history of mental health problems and violence, and that he had been in contact with mental health services shortly before the offences took place.

The response of the government at the time was that the Stone case reflected a broader unwillingness of psychiatrists to address the problem of high-risk offenders with personality disorder by cynically hiding behind the 'treatability' clause of the Mental Health Act 1983 [10]. That is, the profession avoided taking responsibility for dangerous and difficult patients by assessing them as untreatable. Under the 1983 Act, Stone could only have been detained in hospital if 'treatment [was] likely to alleviate or prevent a deterioration in [his] condition' (see Table 1.1). The UK Home Secretary at the time accused psychiatrists of interpreting the law too narrowly. He claimed that it was extraordinary for psychiatrists to only take on those patients they regard as treatable and argued that if the same philosophy applied in any other medical speciality, there would be no progress in medicine whatsoever [11]. Psychiatrists argued that there was

Table 1.1 Criteria for admission for treatment under the Mental Health Act

Mental Health Act 1983	Mental Health Act 1983 (as amended by the Mental Health Act 2007)
Suffering from a mental illness, psychopathic disorder, mental impairment, and/or severe mental impairment; and	Suffering from a mental disorder of a nature or degree which makes it appropriate for him to receive treatment in a hospital; and
It is necessary for the health or safety of the patient or for the protection of other persons that he should receive such treatment and it cannot be provided unless he is detained under this section; and	It is necessary for the health or safety of the patient or for the protection of other persons that he should receive such treatment and it cannot be provided unless he is detained under this section; and
Treatment is likely to alleviate or prevent a deterioration of his condition	Appropriate medical treatment is available for him

no legal provision for Stone to have been taken into psychiatric care simply to protect the public. They also expressed concern that the profession was being used to correct judicial mistakes in relation to offenders who could and should have been given life sentences by a criminal court [12].

The government's response was twofold. First, they amended the Mental Health Act 1983 by removing the 'treatability' clause, so that patients with the new category of 'Mental Disorder', which in the amended Act included those with personality disorder, could be detained on the condition that 'appropriate medical treatment is available'. This brought the Act into line with European Human Rights legislation, which allows the detention of those with unsound mind who pose a risk to others, with no reference to treatability [12]. Under the amended Act, 'medical treatment' included nursing, psychological intervention, and specialist mental health habilitation, rehabilitation, and care for the purpose of alleviating, or preventing a worsening of, a mental disorder, even if it cannot be shown in advance that any particular effect is likely to be achieved.

The second part of the government's response was the development of the DSPD programme. This joint Department of Health and Home Office initiative was introduced in 1999 to address the needs of high-risk offenders with personality disorder [13]. With a joint public protection and treatment agenda, the programme aimed to achieve this by developing services, evaluating them, and developing a broader research programme to address the limited evidence base. The first DSPD service opened in a high-secure prison in 2002, followed by services in another high-secure prison and in two high-secure hospitals. In addition to the high-secure sites, three medium-secure services were commissioned, together with two specialist community services.

Following the decommissioning of the DSPD service at Broadmoor Hospital and the incorporation of the high-secure prison, medium-secure hospital, and community services into the OPD pathway (the service at Rampton Hospital has yet to be decommissioned), the successes of the programme were not as widely acknowledged as its failings. The DSPD programme undoubtedly provided significant investment in a previously neglected population who had had access to little, if any, treatment previously. New treatment models were developed, drawing on the existing criminal justice and non-forensic personality disorder evidence bases, and more than 300 treatment places were created. In an area conspicuously lacking a specific evidence base, funding was provided for a wide-ranging research programme looking at assessment, treatment, cost-effectiveness, and workforce development. Regarding the latter, one of the greatest legacies of the programme is a well-trained, highly skilled body of health and criminal justice professionals with the required competencies to work with personality disordered offenders. The DSPD programme also highlighted the need for non-forensic personality disorder services and likely provided some stimulus for related initiatives such as the National Institute for Health and Care Excellence (NICE) guidelines on both antisocial and borderline personality disorders [14, 15].

Arguably, one of the DSPD programme's strengths was also one of its key weaknesses. That is, although a small number of offenders are responsible for a disproportionate number of offences, focusing on those with the highest risk functionally linked to severe personality disorder is not the most cost-effective means of ensuring maximum impact on violent and sexual reoffending.

One of the most consistent criticisms of the DSPD programme, and perhaps one that was responsible for many of the others, was of the label itself. Misgivings over the concept of personality disorder itself aside, the criteria for severe personality disorder ignored existing evidence regarding the relative contributions of personality traits and criminogenic factors to risk. The predictive validity of the risk measures used raised both scientific and ethical concerns and the concept of a functional link with personality disorder was both vague and rarely sufficiently justified [16]. The concept was based on the assumption that treating personality pathology would necessarily reduce offending, when this was often not the case. As such, it was difficult to ignore the possibility that the invention of this non-clinical diagnosis was primarily to address public protection and the concerns about the management of personality disordered offenders outlined above.

Each DSPD service used a different treatment model, most of which lacked an evidence base in this population. It could be argued that this was a sensible strategy in a series of pilot services to avoid over-investment in one particular model and to provide an opportunity to compare the effectiveness of different treatment models with each other. However, the services were not set up in a way that allowed valid comparison of the different treatment models. This also made it difficult to establish when treatment needs had been met, with the result that the services could form a bottleneck, particularly in the absence of sufficient pathways out of high security. When external evaluations identified that patients spent less than 10% of their time in direct therapeutic activity, concerns were raised that patients were simply being 'warehoused' to manage risk or to compensate for perceived judicial errors in giving determinate sentences to individuals who could be identified as at high risk of reoffending at the time of sentencing [7]. Adding to these concerns was the observation that many patients were being transferred to the high-secure hospital services in the last few weeks of determinate sentences, a practice referred to as 'ghosting'. This undermined several key aspects of good practice with this patient group and resulted in aggrieved patients with adversarial attitudes towards authority and poor motivation to engage in treatment in a way that was likely to result in any positive impact on either psychological well-being or risk.

Unlike the Dutch TBS model, except for the removal of the treatability clause from the Mental Health Act, the DSPD programme was established within the existing UK criminal justice and mental health legal framework. Therefore, entry criteria were clinically defined, rather than legally, and there was no role for the courts beyond initial sentencing.

Independent evaluations of the services were largely critical, in terms of the referral process, service organization, and treatment outcomes [18, 19]. Evaluation of the cost-effectiveness of the assessment process in one of the prison DSPD services indicated that the substantially higher costs when compared with usual prison care were associated with worse outcomes in terms of functioning, quality of life, and aggression [20]. Estimates of the long-term costs and outcomes of the DSPD programme, using decision economic modelling, indicated that the costs of the programme were consistently greater than the value associated with any reduction in serious offending, measured in monetary terms [21]. However, it is worth noting that, despite the significant investment in evaluation of the services and the establishment of a 'common data set' across all services, no high-quality trials were carried out on specific treatments or service environments, and the programme contributed little towards answering the question of what treatments are effective for high-risk personality disorder offenders [22].

OPD strategy

Following the publication of the Bradley Report in 2009 [23] and the public consultation on the OPD pathway implementation plan [24] in 2011, the UK government concluded that the resources invested in DSPD services at that time could be used more effectively in the management of high-risk personality disordered offenders. Rather than any single intervention, the new policy emphasized a whole systems approach, involving a range of providers working in partnership to deliver a pathway of services in a range of settings from high security to the community. All services would be underpinned by the same guiding principles (see Box 1.1). Importantly, the services would be provided within the existing DSPD budget and would therefore be dependent on funds becoming available from the decommissioning of the two DSPD services in high-secure hospitals.

Box 1.1 Principles of the OPD pathway

- An active pathway of intervention
- Shared responsibility
- Predominantly based in the Criminal Justice System (CJS)
- Joint operations
- Whole systems approach
- Psychologically informed
- Mindful of staff and service user experience

The new strategy shifted emphasis from the intensive psychological treatment of a relatively small group of the highest risk offenders in high-secure prison and hospital, to the psychologically informed management of a larger group of high-risk offenders with personality difficulties, many of whom would be under supervision in the community. Services would be jointly delivered by health and criminal justice, with responsibility for the management of offenders being shared between both agencies. However, the overwhelming majority of services would be located in the criminal justice system. A number of key requirements of the pathway were identified, including the early identification of offenders with personality disorder and a focus on risk assessment, case formulation, and sentence planning in the community together with an increase in the number of treatment places within prisons.

In addition to service-specific outcomes, three high-level outcomes of the OPD pathway were identified, namely:

- A reduction in repeat serious sexual and/or violent offending
- Improved psychological health, well-being, stability, and prosocial behaviour
- Improved competence and confidence of the workforce.

Requirements of the OPD pathway

Implementation of the strategy began in April 2012. An estimated 20,000 male and female offenders across secure and community settings met criteria for inclusion in the pathway (see Table 1.2). As of 2017, almost 100% of the National Offender Management Service (NOMS) caseload of approximately 250,000 offenders has been screened against the criteria for the pathway.

In the community, services have been introduced in all probation areas in England and Wales to identify, assess, and jointly case manage offenders

Table 1.2 Entry requirements for the OPD pathway

Male	Female
1. Assessed as presenting a high likelihood of violent or sexual offence repetition and high or very high risk of serious harm to others at some point during their current sentence 2. Likely to have a severe personality disorder 3. A clinically justifiable link between personality disorder and the risk 4. Managed by the NPS	1. Current offence of violence against the person, criminal damage, sexual and/or against children 2. Assessed as presenting a high risk of committing an offence from the above categories 3. Likely to have a severe form of personality disorder 4. A clinically justifiable link between the above

who have been screened. Eight Intensive Intervention and Risk Management Services (IIRMS) have now been established to provide treatment and risk management for the highest risk personality disordered offenders in the community. Mentalization-based treatment for antisocial personality disorder services have been set up at fourteen community sites nationally and is being evaluated as part of a multi-centre randomized controlled trial.

Two hundred and thirty six new treatment places have been introduced across twelve prisons, including democratic therapeutic communities for offenders with comorbid learning difficulties, and existing prison democratic therapeutic communities have been incorporated into the pathway, providing 500 treatment places. Seven hundred new Psychologically Informed Planned Environment (PIPE) places have been created, 552 of which are in prisons and 148 in Approved Premises. One hundred and forty seven prison treatment places continue to be provided in former DSPD sites, and 105 treatment places in one high-secure and three medium-secure hospitals continue to be commissioned.

In addition to service provision, there is ongoing commitment to workforce development, with training specifically developed to meet the needs of staff in the new services in prison and probation. There is also continued commitment to broader personality disorder awareness training for health and criminal justice staff delivered by the Personality Disorder–Knowledge and Understanding Framework (PD-KUF) (see Chapter 2). An independent national evaluation of the pathway has also been commissioned.

Further development of the pathway is dependent on decommissioning of the final high-secure hospital DSPD service. However, it is worth bearing in mind that all of these developments have taken place in the context of unprecedented reorganization in the NPS and prison service and widespread cuts in public sector funding.

Options available

Since 2007, competitive tendering has become commonplace in the National Health Service (NHS) in England and Wales, particularly so in forensic mental health, where secure hospital bed provision has proliferated, in an attempt to seek opportunities for additional income. In higher volume, lower cost prison health services, the tendering process has resulted in robust competitive bids from neighbouring NHS providers. Thus, in the Greater London area, multiple forensic mental health services are often pitted against each other. Within this context, the invitation to bid for elements of the OPD pathway was associated with an impulse to compete, although delivering across a large geographical area and into complex criminal justice systems would have been a daunting task, particularly with the limited resources available. Although such competitive bids from individual providers are often associated with multiple partnerships, these are usually predicated on the model of a lead partner, with subcontracting arrangements and highly specified roles, re-sponsibilities, financial agreements, and performance targets for each of the subcontracted partners. The potential impact of competitive bidding on the OPD pathway for London could have been very significant: a single provider would have struggled to implement a service across all of London, not least because of staff recruitment difficulties; on the other hand, more than one provider, operating independently, could have led to an inconsistent, rather fragmented delivery of the service across the area; and finally, recent experi-ence of the retendering process highlights how much instability is generated by the process, with implications for the transfer of staff, and the demotiv-ation of providers who are exiting the contract.

On the other hand, collaboration between equals—a sharing of roles, respon-sibilities, finances, and performance pressures—offered a compelling oppor-tunity to demonstrate a different way of working within the current climate, and one that chimed with the OPD specification of joint working (see Chapter 4 for more discussion of partnership models). This consortium approach required one of two ways forward. One option was the development of a new company with its own board and financial structure, made up of the partners and linked at 'arm's length' to the participating mental health providers. An alternative op-tion was to adopt a partnership approach in principle and ethos, but one that was legally underpinned by one main contract holder, with subcontracted part-ners, a memorandum of understanding, and terms of reference for the steering group required to clarify the parameters of the relationship.

Our decision was to pursue the latter option, by setting up the London Pathways Partnership (LPP) to bring together four mental health trusts, all of whom had 'a longstanding history and recognized expertise, in delivering effective psychological approaches to complex high risk offenders' (Terms of Reference, LPP, 2015 [25]). This consortium approach was predicated on the model of one main contract holder, largely for ease and speed at a time when the OPD specification was out to tender, but new and untested. However, the partnership ethos was emphasized by placing the LPP steering group at the centre of decision making. For illustrative purposes, an extract of the Terms of Reference is detailed below:

> 'In line with the LPP Memorandum of Understanding and contractual arrangements, each trust has two senior representatives—one clinical, one managerial. The elected chair represents the trust holding the main contract for any particular project.'

The partners were all those who had already demonstrated an appetite and facility for working in the community with personality disordered offenders in London, and who shared the collaborative ethos (although we were rivals in other spheres of service provision!). Together we agreed that our aspiration was to deliver an efficient but effective service across the whole pathway for London, and we would bid accordingly. Our approach was to deliver a service:

- From the community and back to the community
- That was formulation driven
- That was goal oriented
- Overcoming impasse with creativity
- Equipping the offender with realistic goals
- That was consistent across London
- With a relational focus
- Creating opportunities
- Increasing experiences of success.

Our model of care

There were a number of factors influencing our choice of model of care. We were mindful of the literature on therapeutic work with personality disorder (see Chapter 4 for more detail) that concluded:

- There was no superiority of one theoretical model over another in terms of outcomes [26].
- A key ingredient to successful interventions included a single philosophy of care which could be easily shared and understood by all those involved (including the service user).

- The majority of personality disordered offenders do not access or complete treatment (for a range of reasons), and therefore psychologically informed management approaches are key.

We also wanted to learn from the experience of DSPD services (see earlier section in this chapter), which were very institutionally or service focused, resulting in a rather isolationist approach, limited inter-service collaboration, and in inefficiencies in the repetition of core tasks (such as formulation, risk assessment, and treatment content). This meant that our model had to be:

- Sufficiently simple and clear to be applicable across community and institutional settings, understood by a wide variety of both specialist and non-specialist practitioners and meaningful to offenders
- Sufficiently flexible and broad to accommodate various therapy interventions, where appropriate, and not overly restrict the therapeutic orientation and training adopted by a range of psychological therapists.

We concluded that attachment theory was the theoretical model of personality disorder [27] which best met the above criteria, and desistance [28] offered the criminogenic risk model of choice. Our core models are succinctly summarized below.

Attachment theory

Attachment theory, although complex in terms of its biological evidence base and its roots in psychoanalytic object relations theory [29], has tremendous face validity and accessibility for non-specialist practitioners and offenders; it is consistent with the biopsychosocial model, for which there is a growing evidence base; and finally, its relational focus is particularly salient when thinking about sexual and violent offenders with personality disorders [30]. In brief, the offending—as well as relationship difficulties in the here-and-now—is understood as representing either symbolic relationships, objective and real ones, or a displacement of painful emotional states, with patterns of dysfunctional relating culminating in violence, often catastrophic or compulsive in quality.

Offenders with severe personality difficulties usually have both inherited and acquired disadvantages. Genetically influenced characteristics (e.g. impulsivity) interact with the effects of adverse early experiences, particularly experiences in which caregivers fail to provide a sufficiently safe and supportive environment for the child's development. Traumatic childhood experiences are common amongst these individuals, as are multiple disrupted attachments, often including residential care.

Early attachment bonds influence a child's later ability to manage his or her own emotional states, cope with negative or traumatic experiences, and develop his or her capacities for understanding and relating to other people, including the capacity to trust. Negative and abusive attachment relationships in childhood often lead to serious difficulties in adulthood in establishing stable relationships with oneself and others. The difficulties these offenders experience in their adult lives will vary in emphasis, but they tend to have much in common:

- Chronically high levels of anxiety and arousal that cannot be easily managed
- An inability to 'read' other people or think about ('mentalize') others' wishes, beliefs, and intentions; and a tendency to respond to them as if they are abusive, cruel, and exploitative figures from the past
- An extreme sensitivity to experiences of shame and perceived humiliation; this lies behind much serious violence, which becomes a means of controlling others and getting 'respect'
- Poor self-awareness and lack of a sense of identity
- Little sense of being able to influence the direction of their own lives, which are experienced as fragmented and lacking in purpose or meaning.

An example of an attachment-based formulation—albeit a rather brief and simple one—is given in Box 1.2. Mark is a domestic violence offender who has marked antisocial and borderline personality traits.

Desistance

Desistance describes the process of change in which, over time, an offender stops offending and develops a crime-free way of life. The study of desistance highlights the importance of both 'human capital'—the strengths, skills, and resources of the individual—and 'social capital'—the social relationships and opportunities in which those skills and resources can be meaningfully employed—in the effective negotiation of this process. The research also identifies another crucial element: the development of a personal narrative around the process of change, which makes some sense of the individual's past and offers purpose and meaning in his or her development of a different future way of life. The key elements in desistance are therefore building a non-offender identity; developing a sense of personal capability and control; and building relationships that provide emotional and practical support, realistic hopefulness, a valued social role, and a sense of belonging and citizenship.

The utility of desistance as a model is its positively oriented theory, which engenders hopefulness in both practitioner and offender. This is particularly salient for high-risk high-harm offenders who become aggrieved and despondent in response to long lists of risk factors and sentence plans which are historically driven and avoidance oriented. For practitioners, the psychological impact of

> ## Box 1.2 Attachment-based formulation—a case example
>
> Mark has been repeatedly violent to his intimate partners; there is a pattern of him being deeply romantic initially and then increasingly controlling. The victims report Mark picking arguments about trivial matters, as though seeking an excuse to hit them. In terms of background, he was brought up by a depressed and passive mother, and a terrifyingly aggressive father who drank and was violent to his mother. His father always said his mother was the only woman he had ever loved, and they were very wrapped up in each other, despite the violence. As a result, Mark always felt that he and his siblings were ignored. He struggled to manage the tension of wanting to rescue his mother from his tyrant of a father, and yet feeling repeatedly betrayed by his mother's inability to prioritize his needs over his father's. From adolescence, seeking a male role model, he strove to identify with his father, and in doing so, repeatedly sought out relationships in which he anxiously demanded total devotion and attention. This pattern was evident in his offending behaviour, but also in his difficult relationship with his probation officer with whom he was incredibly needy and demanding, but also intensely sensitive to perceived slights.

focusing on the longer-term vision of a gradual process to 'give up offending' is more supportive and optimistic than a failure-driven focus on reconviction. A desistance approach is briefly described in Box 1.3.

It is clear that the process of desistance outlined above is significantly complicated by severe personality difficulties. These individuals face particular obstacles in engaging in a process of personal change, especially in developing a meaningful story of their lives, building a new identity, and forming new social bonds. The disruption to their interpersonal functioning tends to create stress in relationships with others—including staff in the agencies they are involved with—inadvertently increasing risk and inhibiting opportunities for facilitative relationships to develop.

As Fig. 1.1 shows, the overall tasks for the LPP and the delivery of a community to community OPD pathway are to:

◆ *Assist offenders to undertake the key tasks of developing a personal narrative*, through the keyworker/offender manager relationship and, where appropriate, within a thoughtful social environment that encourages reflection

Box 1.3 Desistance approach—a case example

Billy is a forty year old with narcissistic and paranoid traits, and a history of interpersonal violence associated with drug use and association with an antisocial peer group. Having come near to the end of a long sentence for armed robbery, he came to the attention of healthcare professionals as a result of a self-harm attempt after his girlfriend broke up with him. During subsequent sessions with a counsellor, he talked with increasing ambivalence about how 'tired' he was of his lifestyle and image, and his increasing motivation to be a better father to his eight-year-old son than his father was to him. Although there were 'narcissistic' elements to this view of his son, there was also a genuine shift in values around the way in which he wanted to perceive himself. Eighteen months later, after a year in the community, Billy was making progress. Two things were central to this positive state of affairs: first, he had accepted a role as peer mentor with an addictions charity, and this role provided him with stimulation and a necessary boost to his self-esteem; second, his offender manager was supporting him to sort out contact with his children (with the proviso that he remained drug free), and this positively oriented support radically improved their working relationship.

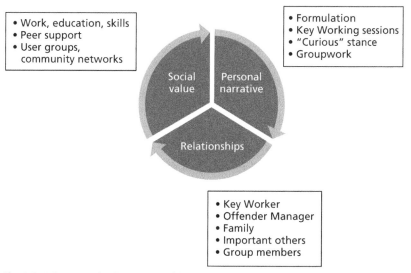

Fig. 1.1 A framework of support and intervention

- *Build their relational experience and awareness*, through the building of a consistent relationship with their keyworker, prison officer, offender manager, and/or psychological therapist, and re-establishing or developing links with friends, family, and other members of the community

- *Gain a social role and value as active and acknowledged contributors to society*, through learning new life and practical skills, developing interests, taking on responsibilities, and building a non-offender identity as a citizen who can contribute to the wider community.

Four years on—where are we now?

In many ways, the OPD pathway strategy can be considered to have been a resounding success. The model is now embedded in every probation area across England and Wales; there is a range of PIPE services in eleven male and ten female prisons, of all types and at all levels of security. More than 30,000 offenders have been identified as meeting the criteria to be included in the pathway, many of whom have been the subject of consultation and more detailed analysis of their presenting issues. The LPP has flourished: the partnership has remained strong, the ethos of collaboration has been maintained, the finances are under control, and the four trusts are, together, delivering across the whole of London community, and into three specialist prison units. There have been huge opportunities for psychological therapies staff in terms of professional development, and recruitment and retention has been excellent with up to twenty-five staff now deployed within the LPP on the pathway. Partnership working with the criminal justice system has had its moments of tension, but relationships have largely been very positive and creative. The LPP has worked with probation and prison services to progress around 600 offenders in the last four years and has encouraged small-scale evaluations to explore the efficacy of the model. The rest of the book will examine all the relevant elements of the model, and highlight the issues in detail.

There has been learning for us, and below we highlight the four main challenging operational issues: the first two relate to the inflexibility of public sector organizations which are not designed to be 'creative' in terms of human resources or finances; the third relates to a universal problem of maintaining performance and impact when shifting from a small pilot to a large implementation; and the fourth is a commentary on the political and social environment which can have a powerful influence on the ability of a strategy to be implemented.

Human resources

Public sector recruitment teams within human resource (HR) departments are understandably conservative and risk averse—staff comprise the main resource of the organization and with them rests their reputation. However, this meant that our attempts for all LPP trust partners to have one shared job description per post, and one advertisement, were disconcertingly frustrated! Partnership trusts 'hosted' staff and retained statutory responsibility for them even though some might have been deployed far from the trust, and this caused difficulties for mandatory training requirements and other core expectations. Trusts took different approaches to the issue of secondment and 'acting up' into new posts. Furthermore, although recruitment and retention were excellent, there were so many opportunities for staff promotion that instability was created with the movement of staff around the LPP services, which again caused consternation for HR departments. An example of how these issues could create difficulties is described in Box 1.4.

Finances

In the competitive environment described above, finances were a focus of scrutiny by the participating LPP trusts. While the LPP steering group forged ahead with their collaboration, and maintained strong trusting bonds, this was not mirrored by our finance managers. The suspicion remained that the main contract holder was 'taking the money'. The reality is that the personality disorder

Box 1.4 Human resources challenges—a case example

Mandy exemplifies the challenges in this area: she was employed by one trust, but went to work in an OPD pathway prison service for whom another LPP trust partner was the lead. This was not a formal secondment—she remained accountable to her host trust LPP psychology lead. After a period of time, she went on maternity leave, which was funded by the original host trust even though she was delivering a service elsewhere. On her return, she successfully applied for a more senior post within the OPD pathway service; this post was a two-year fixed-term position. If it were not to be renewed (supposing the contract for the service would not be renewed), Mandy would have returned to her host trust who retained responsibility for her, but this would have been at the lower grade post.

services are staff-heavy and expensive to deliver, and there are no savings to be accrued. There were additional difficulties in persuading four finance departments all to agree the same level of overheads and costs. We took two decisions: first, all staff would be costed at exactly the same rate across all four trusts, and then each trust would hold the risk of coming in within budget; second, we took the view that transparency was paramount, and we worked hard to assuage anxieties, with the development of a large spreadsheet which itemized every allocation, invoice, and underspend. Any residual monies were scrupulously shared out. It was the main contract holder's Clinical Lead who ensured that the spreadsheet was user friendly and accurate, and the steering group who signed it off each quarter. Interestingly, memories of the LPP's history and structure were limited—a common observation for large organizations—and agreements about staff costing and overhead rates had to be restated annually.

Performance

Despite our best efforts, the rollout of a large community service across London led to uneven progress in different geographical areas and occasional concerns regarding the quality of staff delivery. It has been difficult to ensure that the service maintains the impetus and drive that would achieve an impact comparable to that achieved during the pilot phase. It also became increasingly clear that managers—probation team leaders and area leads—were central to success, in terms of driving outcomes in relation to training targets and the identification of cases. Occasionally, vocal support was not translated into actions. Hard-pressed and demoralized probation officers needed to be tempted into discussing their cases; they, quite rightly, had to be convinced that thinking about personality disorder would reduce rather than exacerbate their workload.

Nationally, the OPD pathway service has been subject to key performance indicators, some of which are quantitative, for example:

- The number of offenders identified in each area as falling within the pathway
- The number of formulations completed, and with what complexity
- The number of formulation-driven sentence plans in place
- The number of staff receiving core personality disorder training.

We were able to monitor progress against these indicators, and in doing so, identified some areas of concern. Staff from both health and criminal justice agencies have variable experience of being at the receiving end of such detailed and immediate scrutiny, and it took time to develop a culture of collaborative self-scrutiny and responsiveness. Our 'traffic light' system—operating mutually agreed indicators of overall performance—enabled us to move forward after a brief period of defensiveness and acrimony.

The prison-based services have not struggled in quite the same way around quality or performance indicators, not least because the staff and the relevant offender group within the services are smaller. Nevertheless, prisons are complex institutions with the potential for toxic dynamics arising out of the mix of disturbed prisoners clashing with a rigid and rather suffocating system of containment. For the prison OPD services, perhaps the biggest performance issue has been the need to evidence a 'value-added' service: that is, demonstrating the contribution of a relatively well-resourced staff team (constrained by rules and restrictions) in terms of the number of hours spent in meaningful and relevant daily activities, and the impact of this activity on hard outcomes such as positive progression into the community.

Organizational issues beyond our control

Unfortunately, one year into implementation, the UK government split the existing NPS into two: high-risk offenders retained by an NPS half the size, and low/medium-risk offenders managed by the Community Rehabilitation Company (CRC) which was tendered out and won by an American private company (https://www.gov.uk/government/publications/2010-to-2015-government-policy-reoffending-and-rehabilitation/2010-to-2015-government-policy-reoffending-and-rehabilitation). The resulting disruption meant that a significant number of staff moved, morale was low, caseloads were newly redistributed, and the OPD pathway had to be reimplemented. A year later, and prison benchmarking was implemented—a government strategy to cut prison costs by £150 million, which resulted in serious staffing difficulties in several prisons, reduced time out of cell, and increased assaults by prisoners on each other and on staff.

These political and social changes serve simply to highlight the relatively precarious nature of service delivery within the public sector, and the near impossibility of achieving a robust evaluation of the effectiveness of the model. A further example is very current and detailed in Box 1.5.

Evaluating our impact

It is a mistake to think that value (for money) equates to services that are cheap. 'Value added' services have the aspiration of deploying limited resources in the most effective manner in order to achieve maximum impact. There is an imperative, during times of economic constraint, to ensure that services can demonstrate they add discernible value. DSPD services suffered from too much being spent on too few with little evidence of social benefit. The current OPD pathway runs the risk of delivering too little to too many, with little evidence of social benefit. The LPP took the view that clinically applied evaluation—delivered by

Box 1.5 Responding to organizational change—a case example

The OPD pathway in the community has targeted Approved Premises (hostel accommodation run by the NPS) which serve the highest risk offenders released from prison into the community. This was a perfect opportunity to target a contained service with the hope of achieving greater impact with limited community resources; training and support with cases were aimed at reducing the community failure rate. However, despite a promising start to this enhanced service, recent moves by the NOMS to reduce the length of stay at Approved Premises in order to better meet demand, the proposed down-grading of the support staff, and the increasingly impossible housing situation have all contributed to undermining any positive achievements from the project.

staff on the ground—was an important adjunct to the more formally commissioned national and London-based evaluations. In particular, larger and arguably more rigorous evaluative approaches run the risk of finding out too late that something has not worked. Evaluation has therefore been conducted at three levels:

1. Nationally commissioned evaluation (National Evaluation of Offender Personality Disorder pathway (NEON)) (2014 to present): following completion of a feasibility phase, this multi-method evaluation will include a process, impact, and economic evaluation of the entire OPD pathway.

2. Externally commissioned evaluation of London (2012–2015): this has been delivered by the University of Nottingham, and comprises a mixed method evaluation of a forty-bed residential therapeutic project in HMP Belmarsh (a high-secure prison in London), and a quantitative analysis of core pathway tasks across London in the community.

3. Local LPP evaluation and audit projects (2010 to present): these have comprised evaluations during and after the pilot phase of pathway development, and include assessments of the impact of training on probation officers, the accuracy of the screening tool as compared to other screening tools, the extent to which prisoners have progressed, and the impact of case formulation on offender manager supervision.

This book

The following chapters have all been written by the LPP leadership team, the exception being the chapter on commissioning where the lead author was one of the original commissioners of the LPP services. Our aim has been to set out the relevant literature, to highlight the pertinent clinical issues, and to account for our decisions and goals accordingly. With the benefit of three to four years' hindsight, we are well placed to review the progress made and to understand the advantages and pitfalls of various options. From an international perspective, we believe the OPD pathway strategy is unique in its conception and in its implementation across a nation; the reader will have a detailed insight into the realities of the strategy.

We commence with a consideration of the staffing and training issues, before moving on to describe the first of the core strategy elements—screening and formulation. The implementation of the strategy in the community is inevitably quite different from the implementation in secure settings, and the subsequent chapters set out these differences, including a description of the therapy elements of the pathway. Service user involvement has arguably taken on a more prominent role in these new services than in other aspects of criminal justice, and we devote a chapter to these developments; likewise, the commissioning model has been central to the success of the new services, and this chapter also provides some reflections from our key partners in prison and probation services. Our concluding chapter is a more personal reflection from the editors, considering the next steps in light of the considerable achievements to date.

References

1. **Morey LC, Benson KT, Busch AJ, Skodol AE.** Personality disorders in DSM-5: emerging research on the alternative model. Current Psychiatry Reports. 2015;**17**(4):558.
2. **Verheul R, Widiger TA.** A meta-analysis of the prevalence and usage of the personality disorder not otherwise specified (PDNOS) diagnosis. Journal of Personality Disorders. 2004;**18**(4):309–319.
3. **Zanarini MC, Frankenburg FR, Hennen J, Reich DB, Silk KR.** The McLean Study of Adult Development (MSAD): overview and implications of the first six years of prospective follow-up. Journal of Personality Disorders. 2005 Oct;**19**(5):505–523.
4. **Crichton JH, Calgie J.** Responding to inpatient violence at a psychiatric hospital of special security: a pilot project. Medicine Science and the Law. 2002 Jan;**42**(1):30–33.
5. **Bortolotti L, Broome MR, Mameli M.** Delusions and responsibility for action: insights from the Breivik case. Neuroethics. 2014;**7**(3):377–382.
6. **Melle I.** The Breivik case and what psychiatrists can learn from it. World Psychiatry. 2013;**12**(1):16–21.

7. Tyrer P, Duggan C, Cooper S, Crawford M, Seivewright H, Rutter D, Maden A, Byford S, Van Marle HJC. The Dutch Entrustment Act (TBS): its principles and innovations. International Journal of Forensic Mental Health. 2002;1(1):83–92.

8. Wong S, Gordon A, Gu D. Assessment and treatment of violence—prone forensic clients: an integrated approach. British Journal of Psychology. 2007;190(49):s66–s74.

9. Darjee R, Crichton J. Personality disorder and the law in Scotland: a historical perspective. Journal of Forensic Psychiatry and Psychology. 2003;14(2):394–425.

10. Maden A. Dangerous and severe personality disorder: antecedents and origins. British Journal of Psychology. 2007;190(40):s8–s11.

11. BBC. Psychiatrists accuse Straw of ignorance. 1998. http://news.bbc.co.uk/1/hi/uk_politics/201795.stm.

12. Maden A, Tyrer P. Dangerous and severe personality disorders: a new personality concept from the UK. Journal of Personality Disorders. 2003;7(6):489–496.

13. Home Office, Department of Health. Managing dangerous people with severe personality disorder: proposals for policy development. London: The Stationery Office; 1999.

14. National Collaborating Centre for Mental Health. Antisocial personality disorder: treatment, management and prevention. Clinical Guideline 77. London: National Institute for Health and Clinical Excellence; 2010.

15. National Collaborating Centre for Mental Health. Borderline personality disorder: treatment and management. Clinical Guideline 78. London: National Institute for Health and Clinical Excellence; 2009.

16. Duggan C. Dangerous and severe personality disorder. British Journal of Psychology. 2011;198(6):431–433.

17. Tyrer P, Duggan C, Cooper S, Crawford M, Seivewright H, Rutter D, Maden T, Byford S, Barrett B. The successes and failures of the DSPD experiment: the assessment and management of severe personality disorder. Medicine, Science and the Law. 2010;50(2):95–99.

18. Trebilcock J, Weaver T. Multi-method evaluation of the management, organisation and staffing (MEMOS) in high security treatment services for people with dangerous and severe personality disorder (DSPD). London: Ministry of Justice; 2010.

19. Burns T, Yiend J, Fahy T, Fitzpatrick R, Rogers R, Fazel S, Sinclair J. Treatments for dangerous severe personality disorder (DSPD). Journal of Forensic Psychiatry and Psychology. 2011;22(3):411–426.

20. Barrett B, Byford S, Seivewright H, Cooper S, Duggan C, Tyrer P. The assessment of dangerous and severe personality disorder: service use, cost, and consequences. Journal of Forensic Psychiatry and Psychology. 2009;20:120–131.

21. Barrett B, Byford S. The costs and outcomes of an intervention programme for personality disordered offenders. British Journal of Psychiatry. 2012;200:336–341.

22. Vollm B, Konappa N. The dangerous and severe personality disorder experiment—review of empirical research. Criminal Behaviour and Mental Health. 2012;22(3):165–180.

23. Bradley KJ. The Bradley Report: Lord Bradley's review of people with mental health problems and learning disabilities in the criminal justice system. London: Department of Health; 2009.

24. **Department of Health, Ministry of Justice**. Consultation on the Offender Personality Disorder pathway implementation plan. London: Department of Health; 2011. http://cipn.org.uk/wp-content/uploads/2017/05/personality_disorder_pathway_feb_11.pdf.

25. **Craissati J.** The clinical development of the London Pathways Partnership. Criminal Behaviour and Mental Health. 2017;27:265–268.

26. **Livesley WJ, Clarkin JF.** A general framework for integrated modular treatment. In WJ Livesley, G Dimaggio, and JF Clarkin (Eds.), Integrated treatment for personality disorder: a modular approach. New York: Guilford Press; 2016.

27. **Ainsworth M, Blehar M, Waters E, Wall S.** Patterns of attachment. Hillsdale, NJ: Erlbaum; 1978.

28. Farrall S, Hough M, Maruna S, Sparks R (Eds.). Escape routes: contemporary perspectives on life after punishment. London: Routledge; 2011.

29. **Bowlby J.** Attachment and loss. Volume I: attachment. London: Hogarth Press; 1969.

30. **Craissati J, Webb L, Keen S.** The relationship between developmental variables, personality disorder, and risk in sex offenders. Sexual Abuse: A Journal of Research & Treatment. 2008;20:119–138.

Chapter 2

Staff selection and training

Chantal Scaillet and Celia Taylor

Introduction

This chapter reviews the literature on the qualities and competencies required for working with personality disordered offenders (PDOs). It considers various staffing models and outlines why the direction of multi-agency, partnership working was chosen—which in turn requires a good grasp of the principles healthy organizations need to apply to be successful. It then explores the needs of staff at all levels for clinical supervision and reflective practice, and the kinds of dilemmas they are likely to bring for discussion. Finally, the chapter examines the results of various evaluation studies of staff recruitment and training, and suggests possible future developments.

Literature review

Staff selection: what is special about personality disorder?

It was recognized from the earliest developmental phase of the Offender Personality Disorder (OPD) strategy [1] that working with this group of people can be highly challenging, both professionally and personally, for the clinical and criminal justice staff involved. Earlier policy guidance [2] had identified certain attributes and competencies as essential: for example, emotional resilience; clarity about personal and interpersonal boundaries; and the ability to tolerate and withstand the particular emotional impact these individuals can have on relationships, both within teams and between services. Although equipping staff with the right skills and attitudes therefore became a key focus of the strategy, surprisingly little was said about how suitable candidates were to be identified and recruited.

It has been known for decades that stigma exists amongst mental health professionals against people with personality disorder [3]. Some of the identified reasons for this include that their behaviour can be demanding, hostile, and tending to invite rejection [4], and perhaps because it is likely to elicit uncomfortable personal responses [5]. Lee et al. [6] allude to the primitive defence mechanisms these individuals tend to use, including splitting and projective identification in particular, which raise 'strong anxiety and difficult feelings in the clinician'. In these circumstances it can be difficult for staff to retain an awareness of the offender's vulnerability, especially when they themselves are experiencing fear, lack of professional confidence, and even a sense of being hated [7].

Unsurprisingly, it is widely acknowledged that staff well-being can be adversely affected by this work, and that high levels of stress and burnout are not uncommon [8]. Some have even recommended that personal health checks should be carried out, both prior to recruitment and regularly post-employment [9]. Aiken et al. [10] in an international study of nurses reported that 42% of the sample described themselves as 'burned out', which is a syndrome of emotional exhaustion, depersonalization, and reduced personal accomplishment that can occur amongst individuals who work with the public in some care capacity. Research shows that probation staff with such clients on their caseload (with a history of violent and/or sexual offences) experience higher traumatic stress and burnout compared to their colleagues [11]. Challenging behaviours and high reoffending or drop-out rates can lead to burnout syndromes, and addressing these issues is paramount, in order to prevent deteriorating health in probation staff. Practitioners can also experience particularly negative countertransference reactions (i.e. unconscious feelings and/or thoughts [5]) to offenders with personality disorder. The alienation that can ensue has been linked to completed suicide by these individuals [12].

In their review of staff in the 'helping professions' (social workers and nurses), Grant and Kinman [13] emphasized the importance of emotional resilience as a safeguard against the stress of the interpersonal and intrapersonal daily challenges. Grant describes how both organizations and individuals need to develop competencies underpinning the development of resilience (reflective ability, emotional intelligence/literacy, social competencies, and social support).

It would seem sensible that what is known about the impact of working with individuals with personality disorder on staff should inform staff selection in services that come into contact with such individuals. The relative lack of guidance on how to achieve this perhaps reflects the paucity of the research literature in this area; such that exists tends to be informed more by experience (including in non-forensic personality disorder services) than by systematically collected evidence. Lee et al. [6] identified a series of qualities and characteristics deemed to be of value by a more-established service and by the Personality Disorder Capabilities Framework [4], a policy document on staff training and development (see Box 2.1). Using a multi-method approach that

Box 2.1 Qualities needed by staff to work effectively with personality disorder

- ◆ Can tolerate frustration and anxiety
- ◆ Able to maintain boundaries while offering flexibility
- ◆ Able to survive hostility without retaliating
- ◆ Can manage internal and external conflict
- ◆ Effective team players, working in a multi-disciplinary team without insisting on strict, professionally determined demarcation of tasks
- ◆ Can assess threats of suicide without anxiety
- ◆ Able to deal thoughtfully with emotional storms
- ◆ Can maintain a robust but responsive demeanour
- ◆ Supportive of reflective practice

Source: data from The Psychiatrist, 36(2), Lee T, Ellingford C, Blackburn S, Bishop E, Ragiadakos N, Elcock P, Bhui K, Selecting staff for a personality disorder service: report from the field, pp. 50–4, Copyright (2012), The Royal College of Psychiatrists.

included role play, an unstructured group with fellow candidates, and a panel interview, Lee et al. [6] found that they were able to appoint staff who later said they felt the process was a valid test of the required skills, and who came to be well regarded by patients in the programme. Including a service user representative was felt to have been a crucial component of the exercise, which ensured that patients' perspectives were represented.

Staff selection: what is special about personality disorder and offending?

Offenders with a personality disorder and other complex needs pose particular challenges to the criminal justice system and to those who work in this setting. For this group of offenders, access to services in prison and in the community is often denied, because they are stigmatized and regarded as more difficult to work with, even compared to non-offending individuals with personality disorder. Bowers et al. [14] set out to determine whether measuring prison officers' attitudes at the time of recruitment could allow the prediction of which candidates would maintain a positive stance towards offenders with personality disorder, over time and exposure. Recruits to the then new

'Dangerous and Severe Personality Disorder' unit at an English high-secure prison were assessed on appointment, at eight months, and at sixteen months, using a previously developed Attitudes to Personality Disorder Questionnaire (APDQ) and a structured interview. Changes in expressed opinions and beliefs were measured, along with behaviours (e.g. rates and types of interaction with inmates), significant events (such as being the target of an assault or official complaint), personal well-being, and performance according to managers' perceptions.

The study found that positive attitudes to personality disorder were associated with better mental well-being, improved work performance, more positive perceptions of managers, and less burnout. The prison officers saw training and education, the support and skills shared between colleagues, and the challenge and purpose of their new roles as positive influences. Negative influences included unclear goals, perceived manipulation by the prisoners, lack of support or feedback, and the sense that they lacked adequate knowledge to cope with the work. While the authors concluded that the APDQ was not suitable for the advance identification of job candidates with positive attitudes to personality disorder, their findings confirmed that these attitudes are malleable over the longer term. They recommended that efforts to create a positively functioning service should focus on the management, education, supervision, and support of staff.

In addition to more formal research and evaluation, there have been a number of narrative reviews of essential competencies for staff working with severe personality disorder. Thus a real interest in the work is likely to be key, rather than what Mothersole [15] describes as voyeuristic motivations, whereby staff are attracted by the thrill of gaining access to notorious criminals. Adshead [16] highlights the capacity to provide a secure base for those with disorganized attachment styles, while Moore [17] emphasizes the ability to provide containment and retain self-awareness, while avoiding high expressed emotion. Finally, Sneath [18] draws attention to the value of a warm interpersonal style, and the resourcefulness to bear hostility without being drawn into retaliating.

What we know about training needs and competences

Policy guidance is consistent in concluding that training is essential for all staff working with individuals with personality disorder [4]. In part, this is because UK pre-qualification education in this area tends to be either sparse or absent. The literature suggests that staff with greater knowledge, understanding, and skills in carrying out the work have more positive attitudes, greater tolerance, and less critical views [14]. They also achieve better engagement, and are better able to communicate a sense of hope that change is possible and realistic.

Wright et al. [19] argue that staff training can increase recognition that people with personality disorder have positive attributes as well as negative ones—a process they refer to as 'a re-engagement with common humanity'.

In 2003, the National Institute for Mental Health in England published a guidance document, *Personality disorder: no longer a diagnosis of exclusion* [2], to facilitate the implementation of standards as applicable to services for people with a personality disorder. The guidance addressed workforce training needs, with an emphasis on developing staff at all levels of experience in the identification, assessment, and treatment of personality disorder. Recommended characteristics of training emphasized a team focus; the need for wider organizational and managerial support; and that the training needs of each person be appropriately targeted, with an 'escalator' of competencies in line with his or her experience and responsive to the needs of the service. This led to the first personality disorder-related workforce development initiative sponsored by the Department of Health: *Breaking the cycle of rejection: the Personality Disorder Capabilities Framework* [4]. The framework emphasized that staff should be equipped with the education and training they need to work with people with personality disorder and that the training should be delivered across a diverse, specialized workforce, as well as to a wide range of specialist and non-specialist organizations such as criminal justice agencies. As such, the framework identifies the specific capabilities required of staff working with offenders with personality disorder at various stages of their careers. It is primarily a developmental tool designed to improve staffs' knowledge and expertise through appropriate life-long training (see Box 2.2).

A subsequent report, the Department of Health Personality Disorder Capacity Plans [20], identified further needs in the development of services for individuals with personality disorder, including workforce development. The report emphasized the importance of staff attitudes and skills within current mainstream services, in ensuring appropriate provision for people with personality disorder. However, it acknowledged that it remains unclear whether or not mainstream health, social care, and criminal justice education programmes provided adequate training on personality disorder.

In terms of competences, although national UK policy guidance and other key statutory documents make explicit reference to developing services that include people with personality disorder, as well as the need for training for all staff working with personality disorder, there is very little guidance available on competencies for staff working outside mental health and/or for staff that are not clinical practitioners. This is in spite of the fact that many non-clinical staff regularly work with people with personality disorder (e.g. probation officers, prison officers). The National Institute for Health and Clinical Excellence

Box 2.2 Principles of the Personality Disorder Capabilities Framework

Training should be:

- Based on respect for the human rights of service users and their carers
- Considerate of how best to reflect service user views
- Aimed at breaking the cycle of rejection at all levels
- Imparting skills in how to foster service user autonomy and responsibility
- Multi-agency and multi-sectorial
- Supportive of team and organizational capacity, as well as that of individual practitioners
- Connected to meaningful life-long learning and skill escalator programmes
- Based on approaches to treatment and care that are supported by research evidence, where it exists

Source: data from National Institute for Mental Health in England, Breaking the Cycle of Rejection: The Personality Disorder Capabilities Framework, Copyright (2003b), National Institute for Mental Health in England.

(NICE) guidance on the treatment and management of antisocial personality disorder [21] stipulates that all staff working with people with antisocial personality disorder (ASPD) should have skills appropriate to the nature and level of contact with service users (see Box 2.3).

Roth and Pilling [22] also outlined a competences framework for psychological interventions for working with people with personality disorder, proposing a set of skills described as 'core underpinning competences'. These core underpinning competences are applicable to any staff, irrespective of profession or setting.

Staff support, supervision, and reflective practice

The need for clinical supervision when working with complex personality disorder is emphasized in several key reports and policy documents. Moore [17] outlines the three main functions of clinical supervision, as listed in Box 2.4.

Alongside clinical supervision, group reflective practice is now regarded as crucial for staff working with personality disorder [3], especially as it provides an opportunity to focus on the complex team dynamics and systemic processes

---

Box 2.3 Staff competencies for working with ASPD

- Frontline staff: knowledge about ASPD and understanding behaviours in context, for example awareness of the potential for boundary violations
- Staff with regular/sustained contact: ability to respond effectively to service users' needs
- Staff with direct therapeutic or management roles: competence in treatment interventions and management strategies

Source: data from National Institute for Health and Clinical Excellence, Antisocial Personality Disorder: Treatment, Management and Prevention, Copyright (2009; updated 2013), National Institute for Health and Clinical Excellence.

---

that arise and which may be destructive (e.g. [23]). Professionals can unconsciously become caught up in enacting disturbed relational patterns that might lead to conflict, splitting, or boundary violations. Taking the time on a regular basis to reflect as a group can assist teams in recognizing how these patterns might be playing out between members (see Box 2.5).

The task: what we did

The overall aim of the OPD strategy is to develop better pathways through the health and criminal justice systems for this group (see Chapter 1 for more detail on this, and the formation of the London Pathways Partnership (LPP)).

Box 2.4 Key functions of clinical supervision

- Formative: contributing to life-long learning and professional development
- Restorative: a space for support, shared understanding, and acknowledgement of the impact of the work
- Normative: focused on good practice standards

Source: data from Advances in Psychiatric Treatment, 18(1), Moore E, Personality disorder: its impact on staff and the role of supervision, pp. 44–55, Copyright (2012), The Royal College of Psychiatrists.

Box 2.5 Benefits of reflective practice groups

- Working more collaboratively
- Translating one's own favoured approach for colleagues
- Being open to constructive criticism
- Understanding the impact of working with this group
- Recognizing when one feels overwhelmed
- Thinking constructively about why a situation went wrong
- Acknowledging when something went well

The primary task for the specialist community pathway staff (both health and Her Majesty's Prison and Probation Service (HMPPS)) was to deliver the specification. Delivering training and consultation sits at the heart of this specification, and therefore staff would need to be able to provide high-quality, evidence-based and psychologically informed feedback, via case consultation and mutually developed formulations, as well as supporting workforce development and identifying personality disorder within the offender population. In delivering the prison pathway, the primary task was to work in partnership with selected staff to engage with a challenging offender population. Core skills were required in interpersonal engagement, an ability to demonstrate curiosity and warmth, and a willingness to reflect on the meaning behind behaviour.

With respect to governance responsibilities, each of the four host trusts was responsible for managing the staff employed to implement the project within their allocated geographical catchment area—that is, a quadrant of London. Staff

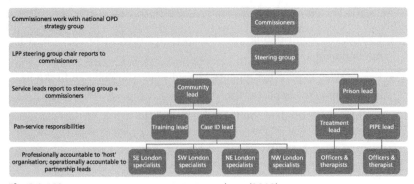

Fig. 2.1 LPP governance structure at start-up phase (2013)

recruitment proceeded in line with the policies of each of the four trusts, although there was some harmonization of human resources policies by a memorandum of understanding, and interested candidates could be seconded from one trust to another. This was coupled with a professional development structure to support staff in further training and development, including identifying and fostering potential future leaders in the field. The governance arrangements involved specialist senior clinicians managing junior psychological therapists, who were responsible for working jointly with their probation counterparts (see Fig. 2.1).

A key finding of the Bradley Report [24] was the difficulty posed by agencies working 'piecemeal' or 'in silos', with no one organization holding clearly identified, overall authority. The report concluded that it is 'the joint responsibility of all the government departments, agencies and organizations [involved] to drive through improvements by working closely in partnership with one another'. Arguably, this axiom is most important of all in the context of services for offenders with personality disorder. The model of criminal justice agencies and health services working in partnership was therefore adopted as a core philosophy of the OPD strategy [1]. It followed, then, that a joint approach to staff selection and training would do much to cement co-operation and effective co-working. All LPP interviews and other approaches to staff selection were therefore jointly conceived and run, which provided a model for successful candidates that would persist into all areas of their work. The application of this approach cannot, however, eliminate the fact that in certain contexts one agency holds primary responsibility—for example, prison staff remained accountable for security and prison operations, while health staff led on the identification of personality problems and formulation.

In the spirit of partnership and collaboration, a model of joint working between junior specialist psychological therapists and non-specialist (but interested) prison staff and probation officers formed the basis of staff selection for the LPP. A fundamental element of this partnership was that of supporting non-health colleagues in case management via a shared partnership and collaborative coaching, rather than assuming an expert position. Embedding junior psychological therapists within probation teams and working alongside probation officers, rather than 'flying in' as experts, ensured a new model of working, in contrast to more traditional forms of delivery in which the National Health Service (NHS) and criminal justice system run in parallel. Cascading information via this partnership provided an efficient and cost-effective model for wider dissemination of training and access to psychologically informed ways of working for whole teams of probation and prison staff, as well as joint working to identify the offenders eligible for the OPD pathway and to facilitate their progression through the pathway.

The model underpinning the LPP approach to managing personality dis-ordered offenders also informed staff selection and the development of staffing structures, in a way that was markedly different to conventional treatment services for such offenders in health settings. A focus on the relational and inter-personal aspects of effective practice with offenders is strongly supported by re-search evidence from the field of psychotherapy (e.g. [25]), which suggests that specific methods of intervention have a relatively minor role in determining success, and that the following 'common factors' are responsible for bringing about change:

- Therapist factors and/or relationship variables (respect, empathy)
- Working alliance (mutual understanding and agreement about the nature and purpose of treatment)
- An approach that is person centred, or collaborative and client driven (taking the client's perspective and using the client's concepts).

Thus, LPP required staff fit for the primary task—a collaborative, relational ap-proach that promotes the development of trust. This has particular significance with PDOs, because difficulties in this area are a feature of the disorder and often underpin individuals' offending patterns. This means that particular attention needs to be given to strategies for building a collaborative relationship. At the same time, focus on the alliance offers an effective way to manage maladap-tive self-views and others' views involving betrayal, abandonment and rejection that underlie interpersonal dysfunction. Other elements of the model include a focus on strengths-based approaches (e.g. the Good Lives Model), where the evidence suggests that the alliance is enhanced when therapist and client agree on set goals and how these goals will be attained [26]. Desistance research sets out to explain factors that support people from re-offending. Individuals are encouraged to build on meaningful personal narratives towards adopting pro-social identities. This is achieved by principally drawing on solution-focused interventions that capitalize on strengths, resilience, and protective factors [27]. Desistance requires social capital (opportunities) as well as human capital (capacities). This suggests an advocacy role for practitioners seeking to sup-port change and underlines the need to target systems beyond the individual offender. This approach to offender management clearly shifts focus away from traditional models of institutionally based treatment provision. The emphasis is thus towards the reintegration of offenders via services that understand the particular challenges of individuals with complex needs. In particular, not only are these individuals subjected to social exclusion, but they are also considered to be at high risk of not managing in the community and re-offending.

The role of the psychiatrist in OPD services has also developed to become significantly different to that in conventional forensic mental health services. Each LPP community pathway service and the prison units all had a small amount of input from a consultant forensic psychiatrist. This was in recognition that disputes and uncertainties about diagnosis can arise, and here a formal assessment by a senior clinician with experience of both mental illness and personality disorder is required. The psychiatrist could also liaise with community mental health and prison in-reach teams, and advise about prescribed medication. Another important aspect of the role was that of making referrals to secure hospital services when required; this is still conventionally done by a psychiatrist; indeed, some secure hospitals do not accept referrals from probation officers.

How to do it

Staff selection

Staff selection should, above all, be based on voluntary applications: requiring individuals who do not wish to work with this group to do so will store up difficulties—if not immediately, then at some future point. The best approach to identifying suitable, interested staff will rely on an awareness of the required characteristics, and first-hand experience of the difficulties they will face. It can be illuminating to place candidates in a group discussion exercise, especially with service users present, to explore styles of relating and to debate carefully constructed scenarios. A service model that relies on a high ratio of junior to senior staff will need to recruit people who can work independently but are at the same time capable of using supervision constructively. A willingness and ability to consider the approach taken by staff from other disciplines and agencies will promote partnerships and mitigate conflict. In view of the enormity of the task of screening all the offenders on probation officers' caseloads across London, this model of collaboration was essential to its completion. The Knowledge and Understanding Framework (KUF) (see section 'Training') [28] was a useful means of sparking interest in potential specialist staff.

The clinical practitioners recruited were usually high-quality psychological therapists who were either chartered or post-doctoral clinical and forensic psychologists, or had equivalent qualifications and experience from a different core professional background. However, the staff team was greatly enhanced when we were able to attract interested occupational therapists and clinical nurse specialists to the posts.

Training

A phased training programme was developed specifically to meet the needs of health and criminal justice staff working in the OPD pathway services. This provided a broad programme of training, ranging from basic awareness to specialist training for staff who had experience in working with personality disorder offenders.

Phase 1: developing awareness across all staff groups within criminal justice

KUF training [28] was jointly commissioned in 2007 by the Department of Health and the Ministry of Justice, as part of the development of a national framework to support people to work more effectively with personality disorder. The key goal was to improve service user experience through developing the capabilities, skills, and knowledge of the multi-agency workforces in health, social care, and criminal justice who are dealing with the challenges of personality disorder. The KUF offers a phased approach to workforce development and, within the pathways services, the KUF awareness (level 1) informed the staff selection process. One of the key successes of the KUF training is the co-facilitation by an 'expert by experience' and a 'worker by experience', which further highlights the importance of service user involvement across the pathways services.

Further training proposed by the OPD workforce development strategy sought to:

- Establish a more psychologically informed workforce, where the meaning of behaviour and pro-social development is seen in the context of a biopsychosocial framework
- Improve the quality of relationships with professional staff, within which offenders can be supported to make positive changes
- Improve the effectiveness and quality of services by developing the capability, awareness, knowledge, and understanding of all staff who work with PDOs.

The above objectives were assimilated into the pathways training ethos.

Phase two: developing skills in the offender management staff group

In keeping with the coordinated joint approach of the pathways model, training delivered to teams was co-facilitated by the Personality Disorder Probation Officer (PDPO) and a psychological therapist. Prior to dissemination, the co-faciitators were initially inducted in a centralized location by the training lead (a senior clinician). This ensured standardization of the material, and aimed to model a coaching and partnership approach when disseminating the training to whole teams.

The learning materials were developed to increase staff participation by incorporating all the elements of active learning in its delivery and approach. The training delivered was informed by a training needs analysis devised to identify training needs for offender managers working across the probation service with a PDO population. The analysis highlighted a number of training areas in relation to the management and treatment of PDOs, namely:

- Developing the workforce and encouraging change in the care of clients to enhance offenders' engagement
- Improving staff's understanding of clients' complex presentations
- Supporting effective risk management plans
- Encouraging psychologically informed thinking and improving staffs' self-efficacy when working with PDOs.

The content of the training was underpinned by psychologically informed ways of working, and linked to staffs' roles within the criminal justice system. The content was based on an existing practitioner guide developed by LPP clinicians [29]. This guide is intended for all staff working with PDOs and provides practical information and advice for managing people whose behaviour can be extremely challenging. It also considers the impact of such work on staff well-being, with suggestions on how staff can protect themselves. As such, the guidance provided the framework for developing the training content as it, in turn, was informed by the robust evidence base on working with this client group. The second edition, which was published in 2015, provides a comprehensive update to the guidance, together with new chapters on working with young adults, working with women, and developing case formulations. This publication has become widely adopted as a framework for the approach of bringing complex psychological ideas into the criminal justice system.

This training not only drew on a range of empirical research into best practice for working with PDOs, but also considered best practice evidence for delivering training to adult learners. Theories of adult learning, known as andragogy [30], informed the delivery of the training materials, as research has shown that adult learners can retain more information when they are able to put their newly acquired skills into practice and are able to reflect on and practice the new learning. The process of reflecting on and making the training meaningful, by linking theory to practice, supports retention of the materials and deepens the learning process.

In keeping with the emphasis on providing a consistent, evidence-based approach to the delivery of the training, materials were printed as a package that included a trainer manual, a trainee manual, and a set of powerpoint slides. The core modules that formed the basis of the awareness training are shown in Fig. 2.2.

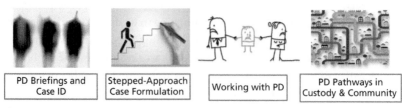

| PD Briefings and Case ID | Stepped-Approach Case Formulation | Working with PD | PD Pathways in Custody & Community |

Fig. 2.2 LPP awareness training

Phase 3: developing expertise in the specialist OPD pathways staff

Not all specialist staff recruited into the OPD pathway were 'specialists' when first appointed. That is, they were not all equally experienced, knowledgeable, and confident in relation to the pathway tasks. Staff in specialist services, however, require a more in-depth theoretical understanding of the origins and nature of personality disorder and offending; of typical complex emotional, interpersonal, and behavioural difficulties; of how to build and maintain the therapeutic alliance; and of the various treatment approaches offered by services. Knowledge of the organizational factors that hinder or promote inter-agency working will also be invaluable.

With these needs in mind, a local training plan for our specialist staff—to include a competency framework for practitioners across health and criminal agencies—was developed. The competency framework had to be suitable for staff that came from diverse training and experience backgrounds, with a diverse range of values underpinning their profession (e.g. health versus criminal justice). The emphasis was on a developmental framework that aimed to highlight opportunities for learning and growth in specific areas relevant to their knowledge, experience, and current work. It was also a tool for enabling staff to set out their objectives against their own identified area of development, as well as an opportunity for peers and colleagues to provide feedback.

Roth and Pilling [22] cite how competence lists need to be of practical use. To achieve this they need to be structured in a way that reflects the practice they describe, and be both understandable and valid. The project-specific competences list was derived by incorporating information from a range of documents—such as job descriptions and statutory guidance—applicable to both clinical and non-clinical staff. A visual representation of the competences was provided via a competences map (see Fig. 2.3). The map organizes the competences into four domains, namely assessment and formulation, case consultation, workforce development, and leadership. Each domain shows the different activities that constitute that area and each activity is made up of a set of specific competences. The required competence

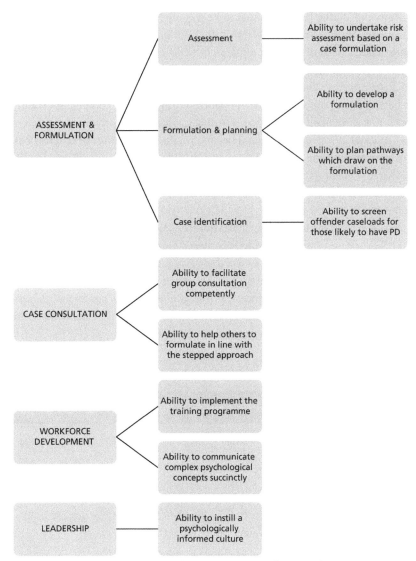

Fig. 2.3 Map of competencies from the LPP competency framework

achievement levels were set in line with the number of years an individual had been in post, so that a newly qualified staff member was expected to achieve a different rating to a person who had been in post for five years or someone with supervisory or management responsibilities. In addition, levels took into consideration clinical and non-clinical staffs' core training and professional development.

Roth and Pilling [22] stress that to be a competent practitioner, knowledge, skills, and attitudes need to be integrated into practice, so that the individual understands not only *how* to implement skills but also what the rationale is behind these (*the why*). With this in mind, the competences were divided into what staff need to know (knowledge and theory checklist) and what staff need to be able to do (skills checklist). It is worth noting that the competency framework was developed as an add-on to those already in place for the different professional groups across mental health and criminal justice. In other words, the basic assumption of the practitioner's attitude and stance was assumed; that is, that any client–practitioner contact was ethical, conformed to professional standards, and was appropriately adapted to the client's needs and cultural context.

In order to fulfil these higher-level training needs, LPP developed a course called 'Working With Personality Disordered Offenders' that was based on the LPP competency framework described above, with due regard to a multi-agency, partnership service model that included staff from a range of disciplines—such as psychologists, probation officers, prison officers, and occupational therapists. The aims of the course, and how they map onto the four domains of the competency framework, are given in Box 2.6.

Box 2.6 Aims of the LPP course: working with PDOs

To develop students' knowledge, understanding, and skills in the following areas:

Assessment and formulation; case consultation

- Explanatory theories/research evidence for how severe personality difficulties develop and their link to offending; for example, genetic influences, biopsychosocial model, attachment theory
- Treatment approaches and the process of desistance
- PDOs' emotional, interpersonal, and behavioural difficulties, in order to match their needs with their pathways

Workforce development; leadership

- Organizational factors that help or hinder effective working relationships, within teams and between agencies
- Application of learning to support the professional development of colleagues

A constant challenge when delivering training to busy staff is that of securing their release from the workplace. Options to address this include intensive, full-time teaching over, for example, two weeks; expecting the bulk of the learning to be done in private time; or holding teaching events at intervals. This latter model suited LPP services better, and was implemented by arranging study days throughout the year, each with a particular theme and each building on the previous study day. Nevertheless, students from the probation service greatly outnumbered those from the prison service, reflecting the difficulty of releasing the latter from their duties. The course was split into two levels, intermediate and advanced, to accommodate students with differing prior knowledge and experience. The Intermediate course ran over twelve study days and addressed competencies in domains one and two of the LPP competency framework: assessment and formulation, and case consultation. The advanced course ran over six study days through the year, coinciding with every other intermediate study day, and covered competencies in domains three and four: workforce development, and leadership.

The teaching approaches included lectures, reading seminars, and interactive sessions, including 'live' practice for intermediate students in presenting cases and deriving formulations, with advanced students overseeing and thus developing their group facilitation skills. An important aspect of the course was the inclusion in the afternoon sessions of experts by experience: ex-offenders with past involvement in criminal justice and/or health-based secure services, who were able to share their knowledge of the realities of life 'in the system'. Their inclusion significantly helped to promote the students' understanding of personality disorder, and to reduce some of the associated stigma and preconceptions.

Supervision and reflective practice

In the interest of meeting these needs, all staff were offered individual clinical supervision by a senior clinician, at a minimum of monthly intervals. Health service staff are accustomed to clinical supervision as a requirement of their professional practice, but probation and—perhaps especially—prison officers approached it, at least initially, with some trepidation, expecting to feel exposed as out of their depth, and hence humiliated. Some expressed fears of 'getting in too deep' with inmates during keywork sessions, especially if sensitive matters such as experiences of childhood sexual abuse came up: officers described feeling 'paralysed' by not knowing what to say, and by a fear of making things worse. Over time, most, however, began to find that the supervision built confidence in their capacity to offer emotional support, and provided an opportunity to develop their thinking. This was reflected in both small ways—such as gradually beginning to call inmates by their first names—and large ways—for example, increased appreciation of the importance of attachments and consistency.

The supervision provided for community-based probation officers was psychoanalytically informed and facilitated externally by experienced psychotherapists. An analysis [31] of feedback forms from supervisors during the early stages of the project highlighted typical countertransference challenges, such as fear, dislike, punitive impulses, or a pull towards over-involvement. They also reflected core organizational anxieties regarding serious further offences, and fears of being blamed by managers and targeted by the media if they should occur. As time went on, however, concerns about major upheaval within the service came to the fore, illustrating the complexity of multi-agency working at a time of rapid organizational change.

One prison-based, multi-agency reflective practice group was able to explore the impact of the new service on the rest of the prison. Common themes were that officers on other wings derided it as a unit for 'nutters', while its staff were referred to as 'care bears' who had 'gone soft' on their charges. Members of the reflective practice group understood that some of this hostility represented envy of the service's higher staffing levels and resources, while acknowledging their widespread fears that the new service could bring a concentration of very troubled inmates to the jail. Themes explored within the team included impulses to 'get rid of' particularly troublesome inmates; the wisdom—or otherwise—of relaxing rigid prison rules to allow for flexibility; who was in charge of what; and the guilt or helplessness many felt upon witnessing deliberate self-harm. As such, a reflective culture is perhaps a less familiar concept to the prison officer transitioning from ordinary prison location to work in a specialized personality disorder unit. In addition, within the prison establishment, one-to-one sessions or supervision can be experienced by staff as a negative, almost punitive, experience. This is especially pertinent in a custodial environment wherein a 'blame' culture is common. A further obstacle to prison staff willingly accessing supervision is the often 'macho' façade adopted by those working in a highly risky, unpredictable, and dangerous environment as a defence against hostile attacks by prisoners. Rewarding and sometimes moving experiences were also discussed, such as contributing to case discussions when the probation officer visited, and meeting a prisoner's children on family days.

In addition to clinical supervision and reflective practice opportunities, LPP staff were invited to attend regular away days to encourage cohesive peer relationships and reinforce governance structures. They were also provided with focused, additional training aimed at equipping them for their roles. The LPP worked with the London probation lead, the prison leads, and the PDPOs to ensure that training was delivered to both specialist and generic probation and prison staff. All probation officers attend regular complex case group consultation facilitated by the PDPO and the psychological therapist. These consultations support discussion around formulating complex cases and pathways planning. In addition to the formal supervisory structures, post-holders are part of well-established and high-functioning psychology departments linked to medium-secure services. This allows for opportunities for peer support and robust professional supervision.

What worked and what didn't

Staff selection/recruitment

Some elements of the model were not as effective in practice as had been expected. The first of these was the health/criminal justice tension within both the community and prison services. It is inevitable that organizational culture played a role in these tensions, as traditionally the health and criminal justice agendas vary in their ethos and primary tasks. The shared values principles of the partnership model, although aspirational, did not always translate into practice. Anecdotally, psychological therapists reported that they were at times met with suspicion and caution by the probation service, attributable in part to the context of the probation service's organizational restructuring. Probation staff job and role uncertainty, heavy caseloads, and administrative deadlines clashed with the need in the initial start-up phase of the project for health staff to embed the model and meet targets. This impacted on the partnership principles, as health staff would, at times, prioritize 'getting the job done irrespective of partnership' rather than risk not meeting targets. Understandably, the priority of the probation service management structure was to meet its own targets, which at times meant inadequate senior management support in driving forward the pathways model. As the model grew, its positive impact on probation staff's competence became more evident and the tensions reduced significantly.

Within the prison estate, the health/prison officer tensions appeared much more to be located within the divergent organizational cultures and underpinning values and principles. These impact on the attitudes and values held by each staff group within these organizations. To illustrate this point, a prison officer's training does not typically incorporate psychologically informed ways of working with disturbed individuals, which is the 'bread and butter' of psychologists. This difference becomes heightened at times of managing challenging behaviours as well as embedding a reflective culture within prisons. Efforts to develop a shared awareness of these cultural differences in order to achieve more effective collaboration include work-force development and the introduction of reflective practice opportunities.

Perhaps inevitably, those who had been working in LPP services for some time gained specialist experience that made them eminently suitable for promotion. This did not create a problem if more senior posts became available within the LPP and these candidates were successful in applying for them. However, it sometimes meant moving between individual trusts within the LPP, which could create tensions, and there was also a limited pool from which to recruit outside of the LPP, as it already included four large mental health trusts with established expertise in managing complex offenders with personality difficulties. Nevertheless, vacancies were almost always filled in a timely manner, including sometimes with external applicants, perhaps due to the widespread interest in services that were benefitting from increasing investment.

Training

Overall attendance at both courses was in the order of 80%, suggesting that the monthly study day structure suited most of the students, despite their onerous work commitments. Study day evaluations showed that the courses were very popular: around 80% of students rated them as very good or excellent, as well as relevant or highly relevant to their work. Free text feedback reflected that students valued the mix of probation, health, and prison-based staff as promoting inter-agency understanding and communication. The Intermediate students in particular varied in terms of their pre-existing knowledge and experience, with prison officers especially having had fewer prior learning opportunities. This meant that certain basic concepts with which others were familiar needed to be reiterated. Aspects of the course were felt to focus overly on the role of the probation officer, as they comprised the largest group.

Evaluation

The LPP model of psychologically informed offender management for high risk of harm offenders with personality disorder was evaluated in its pilot phase [32]. The aim of the study was to evaluate the initiatives taken to develop probation staff's capability to work effectively with this group. The authors used self-report measures to assess competency for working with personality disorder, and to assess team climate. The quantitative measures adopted replicated those used to evaluate the awareness level of the KUF training as part of the National Personality Disorder programme. Participants' professional competency for working with personality disorder was assessed using the Personality Disorder–Knowledge, Attitudes, and Skills Questionnaire (PD-KASQ) [33].

Organizational climate in the probation service was assessed using the Team Climate Inventory (TCI), which is based on the Four Factor Theory of Team Climate [34]. At follow-up, qualitative data were also collected from a subset of Public Protection Unit staff (specialist probation staff) who evaluated their experience of the project. The quantitative measures were administered to 150 probation staff at baseline and at one-year follow-up. The follow-up qualitative data were collected from seventeen probation staff.

The results of the initial pilot found that the probation staff significantly improved across a range of generic and forensic personality disorder-related competencies and there was a significant improvement in one facet of team climate (team vision). The qualitative findings suggested that the primary areas of skills development were in the participants' understanding of personality disorder, as well as their capacity to identify it and develop treatment and management pathways. The results indicated that the project was effective in enhancing probation staffs' overall competency for working with offenders with personality disorder. This included their general understanding, their knowledge of risk-related concerns, their skills in identifying personality disorder and pathway planning, and their perceived ability to access specialist support. However, there was less evidence of improvements in the participants' emotional resilience, and the impact on the overall team climate in probation was limited. Despite this, the weight of evidence suggested this was an effective template for partnership working between the health and criminal justice systems, that enhanced the capability of probation staff to work with high risk offenders with personality disorder. The conclusion was that this supports the implementation of the model to other areas of London and to other probation areas around the country.

The LPP model was evaluated again following two years of its full operational phase [35]. The aim of this study was two-fold: first, to evaluate the rollout of the LPP training approach in developing probation staff's understanding, knowledge, and competency to work effectively with this group of offenders; and second, to explore the relationship between working with PDOs and experience of burnout. As in the pilot evaluation, participants' professional knowledge, understanding, and competency for working with personality disorder was assessed using the PD-KASQ. Burnout was assessed using the Maslach Burnout Inventory (MBI) [36]), which operationalizes burnout as a three-dimensional syndrome made up of exhaustion, cynicism, and inefficacy. These are: *emotional exhaustion (EE), depersonalization (DP)*, and *personal accomplishment (PA)*. An important factor was that at baseline, these measures were administered to 500 probation staff, but at the one-year follow-up, the sample was ninety three. This was attributable in part to a nationwide service reorganization, which saw it probation being divided into the government-run National Probation Service (NPS), and privately run Community Rehabilitation Companies (CRCs). At follow-up, qualitative data were also collected from a subset of seventeen NPS staff, evaluating their experience of the project.

The evaluation found that probation staff significantly improved in their general understanding of working with PDOs; they also significantly improved their understanding of the relationship between personality disorder and risk of violent and sexual offending. However, there was no significant change in terms of improved competency, which the authors postulated might be due to the already high scores on this subscale at baseline, suggesting less room for improvement. In terms of the burnout scales, there were no significant results, which the authors postulated might be due to the confounding impact on participants' scores of the organization's restructure. The qualitative findings suggested that the primary areas of skills development were in the participants' understanding of personality disorder, developing reflexivity, enhancing confidence, and applying new learning to existing practice. The authors concluded that the weight of evidence supports the effectiveness of a joint partnership between the health and criminal justice systems in continuing to provide probation staff with tiered interventions to enhance their practice when working with offenders with personality disorder.

In terms of future direction and research, the authors recommended a longer follow-up time in order to allow for changes in the competency and emotional reactions of staff as, over time, staff develop more expertise and specialized knowledge as a function of their ongoing training. The authors made reference to workforce development with the current focus on developing a competency framework specifically aimed at probation staff whose casework includes offenders with personality disorder. They recommended that future research considers evaluating specific competences against positive client outcomes (e.g. client–staff working alliance; reduced reoffending rates) to identify which aspect of the tiered LPP intervention had the most impact on these outcomes. Finally, they suggested that future research should compare workforce competence and burnout to other outcomes, such as staff sickness, or staff retention compared to a control group in the design of the study.

Next steps

Staff selection

Perhaps the most important lesson from our experiences of recruiting staff is that while knowledge and skills are important, having a real aptitude for the work is essential. This means being able to relate successfully to individuals with severe personality disorder, to colleagues in the same team, and to professionals working in a variety of other agencies.

Conventional application and interview processes, while necessary, cannot also assess candidates for what are, essentially, particular styles of relating to others. In the absence of guidance from research, it is important for creative approaches to be built into recruitment, with a view to exploring how the individual behaves in groups. Applicants can be asked, for example, to discuss carefully constructed scenarios with some service users, which could cover themes such as helpful and unhelpful ways of maintaining a boundary, giving feedback about progress, or whether and how to admit a mistake. The service users should be involved in the debrief, as they often have a 'nose' for how well—or otherwise—they will be able to work with particular individuals. A second important component of the assessment is to gauge how the person relates to colleagues; candidates can be invited to a group interview and asked to debate attitudes and responses to disagreements within teams, or their capacity to consider and utilize differing theoretical models; a rigid adherence to a favoured approach can be a source of conflict. Candidates should always be assessed for their willingness to meet expectations for attendance at reflective practice and clinical supervision. Finally, although not all organizations allow a probationary period of employment, these can be useful in that they offer the best test of an individual's suitability for the work and a formal process of review.

Training

The future of training for working in this field could usefully concentrate on the earliest stages of career development. Ideally, basic training about personality disorder should be incorporated into undergraduate programmes, so that professionals have an early introduction to the field and hence the option to consider specializing from an informed standpoint. This would require incorporation of the subject into pre-qualification training for psychologists, probation officers, and even prison officers. To achieve this, influence needs to be brought to bear on national accreditation bodies. Once individuals have qualified and chosen to work with PDOs, they will benefit from a carefully constructed induction, which focuses especially on developing essential 'soft' skills, such as successful relational styles, and how to form and maintain a working alliance. The temptation to provide long introductory training prior to commencement in post should be resisted: training is best processed and utilized in the context of 'live' examples and cannot be successful in the absence of acquiring experience.

Leadership training is a further area for development: graduates from higher-level courses such as the one described in the section 'Phase 3: developing

---

Box 2.7 Essential leadership skills

- Inspires and motivates others
- Displays high integrity and honesty
- Analyses and solves problems creatively
- Drives towards results
- Communicates
- Builds relationships
- Displays professional expertise
- Fosters a strategic perspective
- Develops others
- Innovates

---

expertise in the specialist OPD pathways staff' will need on-going opportunities for development in order to become the seniors of tomorrow. These could usefully include the development of highly specialist knowledge and skills, for example in the areas of sex offending, domestic violence, or women offenders. In addition, senior staff will need to acquire competence in many aspects of leading teams; this should incorporate not only conventional management tasks such as supervision skills and performance management, but also the ability to think strategically, to delegate, to motivate others, and to build relationships. The most important leadership skills are listed in Box 2.7.

To this end, staff with leadership potential should be identified and provided with extra, individualized input, such that they can develop an increased level of confidence and a personal style of exercising authority. This can be done in small groups to which individuals are able to bring current challenges for debate, in order to facilitate learning from colleagues in similar positions but perhaps facing different dilemmas, and to enhance cost-effectiveness.

References

1. **National Offender Management Service, NHS England.** The Offender Personality Disorder pathway strategy 2015. National Offender Manager Service, NHS England; 2015.
2. **National Institute for Mental Health in England.** Personality disorder: no longer a diagnosis of exclusion. National Institute for Mental Health in England; 2003.

3. **Lewis G, Appleby L.** Personality disorder: the patients psychiatrists dislike. British Journal of Psychiatry. 1988 Jul 1;**153**(1):44–49.

4. **National Institute for Mental Health in England.** Breaking the cycle of rejection: the Personality Disorder Capabilities Framework. National Institute for Mental Health in England; 2003.

5. **Aiyegbusi A.** The dynamics of difference. In J Clarke-Moore and A Aiyegbusi (Eds.), Therapeutic relationships with offenders: an introduction to the psychodynamics of forensic mental health nursing. London: Jessica Kingsley; 2008, pp. 69–80.

6. **Lee T, Ellingford C, Blackburn S, Bishop E, Ragiadakos N, Elcock P, Bhui K.** Selecting staff for a personality disorder service: report from the field. The Psychiatrist Online. 2012 Feb 1;**36**(2):50–54.

7. **Murphy N, McVey D.** The difficulties that staff experience in treating individuals with personality disorder. In N Murphy and D McVey (Eds.), Treating personality disorder: creating robust services for people with complex mental health needs. London: Routledge; 2010 , pp. 6–34.

8. **Freestone MC, Wilson K, Jones R, Mikton C, Milsom S, Sonigra K, Taylor C, Campbell C.** The impact on staff of working with personality disordered offenders: a systematic review. PloS One. 2015 Aug 25;**10**(8):e0136378.

9. **Sainsbury Centre for Mental Health.** Personality disorder: a briefing for people working in the criminal justice system. London: Sainsbury Centre for Mental Health; 2009. http://www.patientlibrary.net/tempgen/22833.pdf.

10. **Aiken LH, Clarke SP, Sloane DM, Sochalski JA, Busse R, Clarke H, Giovannetti P, Hunt J, Rafferty AM, Shamian J.** Nurses' reports on hospital care in five countries. Health Affairs. 2001 May 1;**20**(3):43–53.

11. **Lewis KR, Lewis LS, Garby TM.** Surviving the trenches: the personal impact of the job on probation officers. American Journal of Criminal Justice. 2013 Mar 1;**38**(1):67–84.

12. **Morgan HG, Priest P.** Suicide and other unexpected deaths among psychiatric in-patients. The Bristol confidential inquiry. British Journal of Psychiatry. 1991 Mar 1;**158**(3):368–374.

13. **Grant LJ, Kinman G.** The importance of emotional resilience for staff and students in the 'helping' professions: developing an emotional curriculum. York: Higher Education Academy; 2013. https://www.heacademy.ac.uk/system/files/emotional_resilience_louise_grant_march_2014_0.pdf.

14. **Bowers L, Carr-Walker P, Allan T, Callaghan P, Nijman H, Pation J.** The right people for the job: choosing staff that will adjust positively and productively to working in the new personality disorder (PD) services. Report to the Home Office. London: City University; 2003.

15. **Mothersole G.** Clinical supervision and forensic work. Journal of Sexual Aggression. 2000 Jan 1;**5**(1):45–58.

16. **Adshead G.** Psychiatric staff as attachment figures. Understanding management problems in psychiatric services in the light of attachment theory. British Journal of Psychiatry. 1998 Jan 1;**172**(1):64–69.

17. **Moore E.** Personality disorder: its impact on staff and the role of supervision. Advances in Psychiatric Treatment. 2012 Jan 1;**18**(1):44–55.

18. **Sneath E.** Issues and challenges for the clinical professional. In N Murphy and D McVey (Eds.), Treating personality disorder: creating robust services for people with complex mental health needs. London: Routledge; 2010, pp. 276–293.

19. **Wright K, Haigh K, McKeown M.** Reclaiming the humanity in personality disorder. International Journal of Mental Health Nursing. 2007 Aug 1;**16**(4):236–246.

20. **Department of Health.** Personality disorder capacity plans. London: Department of Health; 2005.

21. **National Institute for Health and Clinical Excellence.** Antisocial personality disorder: treatment, management and prevention. London: National Institute for Health and Clinical Excellence; 2009; updated 2013.

22. **Roth AD, Pilling S.** A competence framework for psychological interventions with people with personality disorder. London: Research Department of Clinical, Educational and Health Psychology, UCL; 2014.

23. **Fallon P, Bluglass R, Edwards B, Daniels G.** Report of the Committee of Inquiry into the Personality Disorder Unit, Ashworth Special Hospital. London: The Stationery Office; 1999.

24. **Bradley KJ.** The Bradley Report: Lord Bradley's review of people with mental health problems or learning disabilities in the criminal justice system. London: Department of Health; 2009.

25. **Smith TL, Barrett MS, Benjamin LS, Barber JP.** Relationship factors in treating personality disorders. In LG Castonguay and LE Beutler (Eds.), Principles of therapeutic change that work. New York: Oxford University Press; 2006, pp. 219–238.

26. **Ward T, Rose C, Willis GM.** 21 Offender rehabilitation: good lives, desistance and risk. Forensic Psychology. 2012 Apr 23:407–424.

27. **Maruna S.** Going straight: desistance from crime and life narratives of reform. Narrative Study of Lives. 1997;5:59–93.

28. **Lamph G, Latham C, Smith D, Brown A, Doyle J, Sampson M.** Evaluating the impact of a nationally recognized training programme that aims to raise the awareness and challenge attitudes of personality disorder in multi-agency partners. Journal of Mental Health Training, Education and Practice. 2014 Jun 3;**9**(2):89–100.

29. Craissati J, Joseph N, Skett S (Eds.). Working with personality disordered offenders: a practitioner's guide. London: Ministry of Justice; 2015.

30. **Knowles MS.** Andragogy in action. San Francisco: Jossey-Bass; 1984.

31. **Wood H, Brown G.** Psychoanalytically-informed clinical supervision of staff in probation services. Psychoanalytic Psychotherapy. 2014 Jul 3;**28**(3):330–344.

32. **Shaw J, Minoudis P, Craissati J, Bannerman A.** Developing probation staff competency for working with high risk of harm offenders with personality disorder: an evaluation of the pathways project. Personality and Mental Health. 2012 May 1;**6**(2):87–96.

33. **Bolton W, Feigenbaum J, Jones A, Woodward C.** Development of the PD-KASQ (Personality Disorder–Knowledge, Attitudes and Skills Questionnaire). Unpublished manuscript. London: Oscar Hill Service, Camden and Islington NHS Foundation Trust; 2010.

34. **Anderson NR, West MA.** Measuring climate for work group innovation: development and validation of the team climate inventory. Journal of Organizational Behavior. 1998 May 1:235–258.

35. **Scaillet C, Minoudis P, Craissati J, Wilson K, Olafimihan O, Grewal J.** The London Pathways Project: assessing competency and burnout in probation services. Unpublished manuscript. London: London Pathways Partnership; 2014.

36. **Maslach C, Jackson SE, Leiter M.** The Maslach Burnout Inventory manual, 3rd edn. Palo Alto, CA: Consulting Psychologists Pr. 1996.

Chapter 3

Case identification and formulation

Phil Minoudis and Jake Shaw

Introduction

The first two stages in the Offender Personality Disorder (OPD) pathway are to identify appropriate cases and construct a formulation. Our approach to case identification uses routinely held case information available to non-specialists working in the criminal justice system. We outline a framework for case identification, including a review of risk and psychological difficulties. The strengths and limitations of this approach are discussed. Formulation is initially used to decide which offenders require a psychologically informed approach to their management. It is recommended without hesitation in the OPD pathway, but the literature questions whether training can improve staff competency, how it is related to treatment effectiveness, and the variation in approaches. We argue that formulation in criminal justice needs particular adaptations, resulting in the London Pathways Partnership (LPP) devising a stepped approach to match the level of formulation to need. The chapter closes with a discussion about future directions in research and practice.

Case identification

Personality disorder presents a significant challenge for forensic practitioners. It is highly prevalent in offender samples, with rates as high as 65% typically reported amongst male offenders and 42% amongst females. Rates in community-based samples have produced slightly lower prevalence estimates. Although to date there has been no prevalence study within UK probation settings that has made use of gold standard measures, studies using screening assessments have estimated the prevalence amongst community-based probationers to be between 40% and 47% [1, 2]. As well as being highly prevalent, personality disorders, particularly the 'cluster B' (antisocial, narcissistic, borderline) and paranoid disorders are strongly associated with heightened risk of violent, and to a slightly lesser extent, sexual offending [3–5]. In response to these challenges, the UK government's recent OPD strategy advocates the implementation of systems to identify all high-risk offenders with probable personality disorder within the criminal justice system (see Chapter 1 for a more detailed discussion of the OPD strategy and its antecedents). It is proposed that early identification will allow proactive attempts to engage these individuals in responsive pathways of intervention based on a psychologically informed formulation of the offender's risks and needs [6].

In order to provide context to this task, the volume of need merits attention. There are currently approximately 250,000 offenders supervised by the probation service in the UK, with approximately 80,000 of these individuals in prison. Previous research by Ullrich et al. [7] found that as many as 15% of all violent and sexual offenders serving custodial sentences of two years and over could be regarded as having a probable personality disorder and could pose a high risk of serious harm to others. Recent projections as part of the UK's OPD strategy estimate that within the current offender population in England and Wales there may be approximately 20,000 offenders classified as high risk of causing serious harm to others with indicators of severe personality disorder.

Prior to the implementation of the OPD strategy within the UK, services offered to this population took a reactive approach to case identification in which potentially suitable offenders were identified through professional referrals and were then subject to comprehensive diagnostic and risk assessments to ascertain eligibility (see Chapter 1). While undoubtedly providing valuable clinical information, the administration of these psychometrics required several hours of time for highly trained staff, prolonged access to the offender, and high levels of offender engagement. As such they are impracticable for use in identifying needs in large samples of offenders, where alternative screening methods are likely to be necessary.

Implementing screening systems for the identification of personality disorder in offenders holds a number of potential benefits. First, offenders with severe personality disorders may present with elevated risk profiles but struggle to derive benefit from mainstream offending behaviour programmes.

Second, they may present with low levels of readiness to engage in rehabilitative interventions. Sentence planning for these offenders is therefore likely to be more complex, requiring a more protracted focus on engagement and motivational work, and may also require access to specialist treatment services. Identifying these individuals early in their sentences allows the targeting of specialist support in a planned and sequenced manner, based on a formulation of the offender's needs. Given that offenders with personality disorder are disproportionately represented amongst samples of repeat violent offenders, early identification and intervention is also likely to hold promise as a means of enhancing public protection [8]. Unfortunately, experience from the UK has illustrated that too often the needs of these offenders are identified inconsistently and often at a late stage in their sentence, when they are subject to pre-release risk assessments. This is compounded by the fact that offenders with personality disorder often present with challenging institutional behaviour and may have low levels of motivation to enter treatment [9]. Identifying outstanding risk and treatment needs at a late stage in these individual's sentences is likely to exacerbate feelings of grievance and associated engagement difficulties, resulting in poorly timed referrals to treatment services and unnecessary delays in release [10]. Proactive, early identification should therefore allow attempts to be made to engage these individuals in their intervention pathways from the earliest point in their sentence, thereby making the best use of their time in custody.

Third, systematic screening of complete offender samples minimizes the potential for practitioner bias in rates of identification, ensuring that all cases are considered, not just those with more dramatic or help-seeking presentations. This should allow more effective targeting of often scarce resources towards those with the highest level of need, thereby enhancing the likelihood of positive outcomes. Given these potential benefits, attention is now turned to the means through which this task can be achieved.

Options available

To the current authors' knowledge there is little to no international evidence relating to the implementation of large-scale systems for screening high-risk offenders with personality disorder. There is, however, a wide range of existing screening tools for assessing the possible presence of personality disorders which are currently available to forensic practitioners. These include those that follow nosological systems of categorical diagnosis, such as the International Personality Disorder Examination Screening Questionnaire [11], those that assess individual syndromes, such as the Antisocial Personality Questionnaire [12], and generic measures, such as the Standardized Assessment of Personality Disorder—Abbreviated Scale (SAPAS) [13]. A detailed discussion of these methods is beyond the scope of this chapter, and interested readers are referred to a comprehensive review by Furnham et al. [14]. However, despite the proliferation of existing psychometrics, there are a number of potential limitations with their use when screening for high-risk offenders.

First, the majority of these tools make use of self-report methods, which require the active participation of the individual being assessed and are reliant on their insight and willingness to divulge negative personal characteristics.

Although several self-report personality disorder measures have been subject to forensic validation with adequate psychometric properties [15], their ability to identify antisocial personality disorder (ASPD) characteristics is less consistently evidenced [16]. Furthermore, there is likely to be a tendency in certain forensic settings for respondents to be motivated to produce socially desirable responses and 'fake good', leading to false negative results. This may be especially likely in pre-sentence or pre-release settings. In contrast, there may be a tendency amongst certain highly distressed, help-seeking individuals (a presentation often observed in borderline personality disorder) to produce response profiles that may exaggerate the true level of the underlying pathology. Therefore, any attempt at implementing wide-scale screening using self-report methods would need to consider how to respond to concerns about the validity of the results or non-compliance with the screening process.

Second, research has not demonstrated a reliable association between self-reported personality disorder and elevated risks of violence in forensic samples [1, 17]. This last point is important, and is elaborated upon in the section 'Why we chose our approach'. If the purpose of screening is to identify high-risk offenders with personality disorder, then this needs to be borne in mind.

A further complication when considering the use of self-report methods is the geographical location of offenders, who will reside within a diverse range of settings, ranging from their own homes in the community, to probation hostels, to prisons and secure hospitals.

Lastly, when initially implementing any process for systematically screening suitable offenders, one needs to consider methods for identifying those who are already in the system, currently serving sentences, and those who are sentenced going forward.

It should be apparent from this brief discussion that if using self-report methods, arranging access to all offenders in the criminal justice system, while not impossible, would pose considerable logistical difficulties.

An alternative approach, which overcomes these logistical difficulties, is to implement a file-based screen, using existing case material to identify proxy variables which act as indicators of personality disorder. Although conceptually distinct, the criminogenic needs identified in many existing risk assessment frameworks can be regarded as variants of stable underlying trait dispositions. As such, they can provide valuable information about the possible presence of personality disorder.

An example of this approach is the screen for antisocial personality features, which exists within the Offender Assessment System (OASys). OASys is an example of the structured professional judgement approach to risk assessment. It is the primary risk management tool used by staff within Her

Majesty's Prison and Probation Service (HMPPS) in the UK to assess the risk posed by an individual offender and his or her offence-related needs. It is a broad-based assessment, which contains summary information on all relevant aspects of an offender and his/her history. The assessor is guided to consider a range of domains, which have an empirical association with risk of future offending. It is used to assess and manage over 250,000 offenders each year in England and Wales [18] and comprises an assessment of both static (fixed) and dynamic (changeable) factors. It contains within it three actuarial assessments of offending risk, which provide a percentage likelihood of reconviction as well as a risk category. These three assessments include the Offender Group Reconviction Scale (3rd edition) (OGRS3), comprised of static variables, and the OASys General Offending Predictor (OGP), which also includes a number of dynamic items. OASys also contains an actuarial violence risk assessment called the OASys Violence Predictor (OVP), comprising both static and dynamic items. Offenders assessed using OASys are also designated a separate summary risk level called the OASys Risk of Serious Harm (RoSH) classification. This is the offender manager's professional judgement of the likelihood of the individual causing serious harm, after all other factors in the assessment (including OGRS3, OVP, and OGP) have been considered.

The OASys assessment also contains within it a ten-item screen for anti-social personality features, using items derived from the broader assessment. The screen has previously demonstrated a strong association with measures of sexual and violence risk and been shown to predict community failure amongst community-based sexual offenders [1, 19]. It has also demonstrated a moderate, statistically significant correlation with total scores on the Hare Psychopathy Checklist-Revised (PCL-R) amongst UK prisoners in personality disorder treatment services (personal communication, Jenny Tew, National Offender Management Service, 13 September 2011). The OASys items contained within the screen are presented in Box 3.1.

Although the items within the screen bear considerable resemblance to psychopathic personality traits, it is evident that they were not originally designed for this task, and to date the screen has not been subject to an empirical validation. The extent to which assessors are considering the presence of persistent and pervasive traits when rating the dynamic items in the scale, or more transient offence-related states, is therefore unknown.

However, Bui et al. validated an additional method of screening for ASPD using OASys [20]. They found that their method obtained an Area Under the Curve (AUC) of 0.72 when compared to 'gold standard' diagnostic assessments of personality disorder using the Structured Clinical Interview for Diagnosing DSM-IV personality disorders (SCID-II). The validation sample comprised

Box 3.1 The OASys ASPD screen

- One or more convictions aged under 18 years
- Offences include violence/threat of violence/coercion
- Offences include excessive violence/sadism
- Does the offender fail to recognize the impact of his or her offending on the victim/community/wider society?
- Over-reliance on friends/family/others for financial support
- Manipulative/predatory lifestyle
- Reckless/risk-taking behaviour
- Childhood behavioural problems
- Impulsivity
- Aggressive/controlling behaviour

1,396 adult male offenders (the prisoner cohort) serving determinate sentences of a minimum of two years for sexual or violent offences. In accordance with DSM-V criteria, the method requires identification of three out of five indicators of conduct disorder and four out of five markers of adult antisocial behaviour. The variables that comprise the Bui et al. screen are presented in Box 3.2.

Subsequent research carried out by Shaw and Edelmann [21] using this method demonstrates its utility in identifying a cohort of offenders at particularly high risk of failing to make progress on community-based offending behaviour programmes. More specifically, the Bui et al. screen was found to be the strongest predictor of both attrition and low facilitator ratings of engagement and understanding amongst 571 offenders referred to community-based cognitive skills and anger management programmes. What is notable about this study is that the measure outperformed actuarial risk assessments, including the OGP and OVP, demographic factors, and the presence of learning difficulties in predicting these outcomes.

There is therefore evidence that file-based screens, drawing on criminal history and criminogenic need variables, can be used to screen for ASPD and can achieve acceptable psychometric properties. These screens have shown predictive validity in that they are able to identify a group of offenders who are at heightened risk of both community failure and making limited progress in accredited offending behaviour programmes. Of course, the major limitation to the aforementioned screens is that they only screen for antisocial personality

Box 3.2 Bui et al. OASys ASPD screen

Conduct disorder criteria

◆ Age at first conviction under 14

◆ Age at first contact with police under 14

◆ Court appearances under the age of 18

◆ Serious problems with school attendance

◆ Childhood behavioural problems

Adult antisocial criteria

◆ Convictions for burglary

◆ Convictions over the age of 18

◆ Illegal earnings are a source of income

◆ Easily influenced by criminal associates

◆ Serious problems with impulsivity

features and are unlikely to allow the identification of traits outside the anti-social spectrum.

Given that the task at hand is to identify those offenders with personality disorder who present a high risk of serious harm to others, the relationship between personality disorder and risk of sexual and violent offending also merits discussion. At a diagnostic level, the relationship is strongest for the cluster B diagnoses within the DSM-V and ASPD in particular [22]. However, other personality disorder diagnoses hold a less robust association with recidivism, and some, such as the avoidant and obsessive-compulsive, may even be protective [5]. Where personality disorder is associated with an elevated risk of sexual and violent offending, this is due to a complex interaction between multiple causal mechanisms, including variables at the societal, relational, and individual levels [23]. At the individual level these are likely to include the presence of core personality traits associated with a risk of interpersonal violence, such as emotion dysregulation, impulsivity, narcissism, and paranoid thinking [24]. These core personality traits, their developmental antecedents and their secondary behavioural manifestation overlap considerably with variables that are known to be associated with an increased risk of sexual and violent offending. Accordingly, offenders with personality disorder are likely to present with multiple criminogenic needs, which are likely to aggravate the risk profile further. These may include difficulties with substance misuse, employment, and intimate and peer relationships, and histories of childhood adversity, as well as comorbid mental illnesses associated with serious offending (such as bipolar disorder, attention deficit hyperactivity disorder (ADHD), and psychotic illnesses).

Why we chose our approach

It should be apparent from the preceding discussions that although a range of potential methods can be implemented to identify high-risk, high-harm offenders with personality disorder, all have limitations. In order to develop a system for identifying this group of offenders, the current authors compared the results of various methods, while working alongside offender managers in public protection units in the UK [25]. Three methods of identifying suitable cases for intensive, psychologically informed case management were trialled. The first was via offender manager initiated referrals, in which referrals were brought for consultations based entirely on the offender manager's concerns about the case and desire for specialist input. The second was via an analysis of all cases scoring highly on the the OASys personality disorder screen. The third method trialled was a combination approach using an initial review of risk indicators alongside a broader review of case material, aiming to identify more diverse (primarily cluster B) pathology, not limited to antisocial.

It was found that the probation officer-initiated referrals resulted in a proportion of appropriate and highly complex cases being referred, often with quite severe and diverse personality disturbance (primarily including borderline paranoid and schizoid presentations). These offenders typically had committed very serious offences, a higher likelihood of having sexual and physical abuse histories, a history of suicide attempts and self-harm, and prior contact with mental health services. However, these cases were less likely to be classified as a high likelihood of violent or sexual recidivism according to actuarial risk predictors, although their histories clearly demonstrated a capacity for causing serious harm. They were also likely to be serving lengthy custodial sentences and were therefore less likely to be at imminent risk of further offending. In contrast, however, the antisocial sample identified by the OASys personality disorder variables was less likely to present with these comorbidities and have histories of severe psychosocial adversity, but were higher risk on static measures of general and violent offending risk (the Risk Matrix 2000/V and the OGRS3) [25]. This illustrates a rather crude distinction between offenders with personality disorder who could be considered as high harm, high pathology but with lower likelihood of further offending and those offenders whose offences are of moderate harm but with high frequency and high likelihood of further offending.

Subsequently, Shaw et al. [1] trialled the use of the SAPAS as a means of identifying personality disorder in a UK probation context. The measure was administered to a representative sample of 447 offenders serving community sentences. Demographic and risk data as well as scores on the OASys personality disorder screen were collected. It was found that 40.3% of the sample met criteria for personality disorder according to the SAPAS, with 15.1% meeting the cutoff on the OASys screen. Contrary to expectations, there was little overlap between the subgroups of offenders identified by these two methods. While the SAPAS identified a cohort that was more likely to have a history of self-harm or suicide attempts and experience difficulties coping, the measure bore no relation to actuarial assessments of general and violent offending risk. More recently, Pluck et al. [2] also administered the SAPAS to 174 probationers in the UK alongside measures of alcohol and illicit substance misuse. They found that 47% of the probation cases screened met personality disorder criteria according to the SAPAS, with these offenders having a significantly elevated likelihood of having substance misuse problems. However, in parallel to the findings of Shaw et al. [1], cases identified by the SAPAS were not rated as significantly higher risk of recidivism than the broader probation caseload.

Taken together, this body of research illustrates that in order to adequately identify those offenders with personality disorder who present the highest risks of causing serious harm, it is not sufficient to assess for the generic presence of personality disorder, especially if using self-report measures. Instead, it is important to attempt to identify those personality attributes with a demonstrated association with serious offending (notably cluster B and paranoid personality disorders) and also to review the broader risk profile, as determined by standardized, structured risk assessment frameworks. In light of this, the current authors have developed and implemented an integrated approach to screening for high-risk, high-harm offenders with personality disorder, which allows practitioners to make use of multiple sources of information, while bearing in mind their likely limitations. The framework is presented in Table 3.1.

The intention within this approach is to provide structure to the screening process, using a decision-making algorithm, while enabling practitioners to use clinical judgement when scoring the individual items. It is proposed that practitioners first review indicators of risk of causing serious harm to others, before subsequently considering the possible presence of personality disorder.

The review of risk indicators is structured to comply with the requirements of the OPD programme; that interventions be provided to those offenders with suspected personality disorder who present a high risk of violent or sexual offence repetition and as presenting a high or very high risk of serious harm to others. The algorithm therefore aims to ensure that both high-seriousness and high-frequency offenders are included, as long as they have a history of serious interpersonal violence and/or sexual offences. Although the OASys RoSH

Table 3.1 An algorithm for screening for high-risk, high-harm offenders with personality disorder

Step 1: Check risk level	Check one or more boxes to progress
a. Indeterminate sentence	
b. Determinate sentence for sexual or violent offence Or women only—any sentence type for an offence of violence, criminal damage, sexual (not economically motivated), or against children	
c. OASys RoSH rating high or very high	
d. Medium RoSH, but with past sexual or violent offences	
e. Women only: high risk of further offences of violence, criminal damage, sexual (not economically motivated), or against children	
Step 2: Check for personality disorder indicators	**Check one or more boxes to progress**
a. 7 + OASys ASPD items endorsed	
b. Childhood difficulties—physical, sexual, emotional abuse and neglect, and/or childhood behavioural problem	
c. History of mental health difficulties—that are persistent over time. Isolated incidents related to adjustment problems would not be scored here	
d. Self-harm/suicide attempts—isolated incidents would not be scored here	
e. Severe challenging behaviour—may include making frequent written complaints, adjudications for violence, failures while under supervision, dismissal from treatment provision	
Step 3: Screen in/out	
Step 1 (a–d) + Step 2 (a)	**Screen in**
Step 1 (a–d) + Step 2 (b + (1× c–f))	**Screen in**
Step 1 (a–d) + Step 2 (2× c–f)	**Screen in**

assessment was used as a risk indicator, it was not relied upon exclusively. This was due to concerns about the consistency of its application resulting in the possibility that eligible cases would be missed if relying on it alone [26]. Accordingly, a number of additional risk indicator variables were included, including a review of the individuals' history of serious sexual and violent offending as well as their current sentence. Indeterminate sentences were included as a marker of offence seriousness. These included life sentences and the (now abolished) Indeterminate Sentences for Public Protection (IPP). With these sentences the offender can apply to the Parole Board to be considered for release once a minimum sentence period has expired. The onus is on the offender to persuade the Board that they present a low enough risk to be safely released. Consistent with the guidance in the OPD programme, female offenders are included with lower seriousness offences due to the smaller numbers of females in the criminal justice system that are classified as high risk of serious harm to others.

The assessment of personality disorder is completed via a review of antisocial traits within the OASys personality disorder screen and the offender's history of self-harm, or suicide attempts, given the robust association between cluster B pathology and raised risk of violence. For the OASys personality disorder screen, the threshold of seven or more items endorsed was used, to ensure a broad range of traits were present and also to remain consistent with previous research which has been conducted on this screen. Having a history of significant childhood adversity was included due to the association between childhood maltreatment and later personality disorder, and the association between this maltreatment and later risk of violence [27]. Having a history of mental health difficulties was also included. This item takes a broad perspective and may include the results of completed personality assessments, a diagnosis of personality disorder in the case file, relevant childhood diagnoses (such as conduct disorder or ADHD), or a history of contact with mental health services, which suggests possible personality disorder (such as frequent emotional crises). Lastly, severely challenging behaviour was included to allow for an evaluation of patterns of non-compliance and oppositional behaviour which may indicate severe personality pathology. This might include, for example, having a history of multiple breaches or recalls while under community supervision, numerous custodial adjudications for violence, protracted or frequent periods in segregation, very frequent or diverse offending, or persistent and highly antagonistic behaviour. For all items, assessors are guided to ensure that evidence is sufficiently persistent and pervasive to suggest pathological personality traits.

As the intention of the screen is to identify severe forms of personality disorder, a minimum of two personality disorder indicators is required, except where the predominant presenting pathology is antisocial, given the relationship between antisocial personality traits and risk. Although the algorithm is essentially a file-based screen, it is one that does require a degree of professional judgement, and a clinical override was permitted with regard to the presence of personality pathology where the results appeared contradictory or were inconclusive. The process requires that the assessing professional reviews all available information, which may include personal knowledge of the offender as well as information contained in the file, and scores each item according to his or her knowledge of the case. Although a working knowledge of personality disorder is required in order to implement the screen as intended, it is intended to be used by non-mental health specialists. It is also important to emphasize that this screening process is non-diagnostic and that those being identified are considered likely to present with persistent and pervasive psychological difficulties (which may suggest personality disorder) and a high risk of harm to others.

It is acknowledged that this approach to screening is limited by the available information, and where this is limited or of poor quality the results of screening using this approach are likely to be compromised. However, the algorithm does not preclude the implementation of other approaches (such as self-report screening methods), which can be assimilated within the screening process (and may be coded under the *Mental Health Difficulties* item). Moreover, the intention is to guide the assessing professional to consider all available information and ultimately to take a view on the likely presence of severe personality disorder and high risk of causing serious harm to others, keeping all of this in mind.

What worked and what didn't

Despite working across a wide geographical area and with a diverse staff group, internal audits by the LPP have illustrated that the algorithm approach can be completed consistently, with 93% of cases audited demonstrating appropriate indicators of high risk of harm and 94.5% of cases having the stipulated indicators of personality disorder [28]. In addition, the algorithm has been advocated for use across the OPD pathway nationally and is included in Ministry of Justice guidance on working with offenders with personality disorder [29]. Of course, it is acknowledged that the algorithm approach has not yet been subject to empirical validation, and so the extent to which it accurately identifies individuals who would meet diagnostic criteria according to gold standard measures is not known. A possible improvement to the current method would of course be to implement the recently validated Bui et al. method in place of the current OASys personality disorder screen, which does at least have demonstrated psychometric properties for identifying ASPD.

An informal telephone survey of clinical leads across the national OPD pathway (personal communication, Jackie Craissati, Consultant to the OPD programme, 11 July 2016) suggested that although there was general endorsement for the utility of the case identification screen, a number of limitations were highlighted. First, it was suggested that, given the inclusion of variables associated with cluster B personality pathology, the screen may be less reliable for assessing cluster C personality disorders, which are common amongst child sexual offenders. Second, it was suggested that those offenders who present with schizoid presentations, who may have committed very serious or unusual offences, may also be less reliably identified. These offenders may not present with persistent challenging behaviours or emotional instability which would result in positive identification. It was reported that this was a dominant reason that a clinical override was used in the screening process.

In addition, data obtained by the Commissioning Support Unit within the OPD programme [30] have revealed considerable variation between probation areas in terms of the proportion of cases screened positively (from 25% in Wales to 47% in the Midlands). Although some variability in the underlying morbidity levels is to be expected, it is likely that these variable identification rates may reflect variability in screening practices. For example, outcomes of a related approach to screening for personality disorder in a probation context as part of the OPD pathway have been reported by Nichols et al. [31]. These authors reported a similar approach to screening for personality disorder in a community probation context. The screening algorithm employed was similar to that employed across London and also used the OASys personality disorder screen but did not include an initial filter for risk of serious harm. It also included a greater emphasis on pervasive symptomology and less of a focus on antisocial traits specifically. This screening strategy resulted in a positive identification rate of 18% of the total caseload, which was similar to the proportion identified in the London projects. However, the sample comprised more community cases, with only one-third in custody (approximately 35%, compared to approximately 75% in London) and nearly half classified as medium risk of causing serious harm to others in OASys (49.2% of the sample).

Of course, focusing more on community cases makes sense if one is prioritizing the goal of attempting to reduce community failure and serious community-based recidivism. However, it also needs to be borne in mind that predicting serious repeat offending is notoriously difficult, given the limitations of current risk assessment frameworks and the very low base rates of this behaviour. This is illustrated by research by Craissati and Sindall [32] who investigated the characteristics of 94 offenders who committed serious further offences (SFOs) while under probation supervision. They found that the majority of offenders committing SFOs were in fact classified as medium risk in OASys at the time of the offence. However, it was also noted that these cases were essentially indistinguishable from the broader probation caseload in all variables investigated. It should therefore be clear that attempts to identify those medium-risk cases who are at heightened risk of committing further serious offences is fraught with difficulty and will inevitably result in high numbers of false positive identifications. Ultimately the question of whether to target community- or institutionally-based offenders and those of lower risk classifications is likely to be a matter of resources.

A number of learning points have arisen through the implementation of case identification systems as part of the OPD strategy. First, the systematic screening has highlighted the needs of offenders with personality disorder, which has raised a number of difficulties with regard to how these needs may be best met. Also, the sheer volume of cases identified through screening has vastly outweighed the available spaces in specialist treatment and psychosocial support services, despite the recent rapid expansion of these services in the UK. This has the potential to raise the offenders' expectations of their needs being addressed, and to also raise the professionals' expectations that the needs must be addressed by specialist services before progression can be considered. This is particularly the case for younger adult offenders, who are disproportionately represented within the OPD caseload. For example, in the London area alone there are currently approximately 700 prisoners under the age of 21 screened into the pathway, although nationally there are only seventy specialist treatment spaces in UK prisons for offenders aged 18–21.

Second, it has become apparent that despite broadly proportionate rates of identification across ethnic groups, not all groups access services at similar rates. Previous research, which has largely sampled service users accessing personality disorder-related treatment, has illustrated that black and minority ethnic offenders are under-represented in these samples [33]. It would therefore be expected that using a systematic approach to screening for personality disorder would be likely to produce much more representative rates of identification in these groups, which may subsequently assist in facilitating access to treatment services. A recent internal audit by the LPP of the risk and demographic profiles of 5,923 high-risk, high-harm offenders with personality disorder identified that offenders who were classified as black or mixed race were proportionally represented when compared to the broader probation caseload [28]. Despite this, there were some notable differences in the presentation of the different ethnic groups within the sample. Notably, black and mixed-race offenders with suspected personality disorder were significantly more likely to be classified as high risk by their offender managers. Whether this represents true differences in the presence of risk-related needs or prejudicial risk assessment practices is not known. In addition, black and mixed-race offenders were significantly less likely to have a history of self-harm or making suicide attempts than their white counterparts. This same audit identified that there was no bias in rates of referrals being made to specialist treatment services according to ethnicity. However, the recent outcome evaluation of the LPP community services [34] identified that these offenders were significantly less likely to enter into treatment services than their white counterparts. Although the reasons for this impasse are not clear, what is clear is that there are questions still to be answered about how best to meet the needs of this population, which is given increasing emphasis due to the high level of need being identified.

Third, there is a need to ensure that the results of screening are recorded and communicated accurately and in a way that avoids the use of definitive diagnostic labels. This is especially important given the potentially stigmatizing nature of the label of personality disorder and the perceived association with elevated risk. Given that the overall aim of implementing any screening programme is ultimately to support offenders with these difficulties in accessing support, which will help reduce risks and enhance their well-being, it is important that the label is not used in a way that may hinder engagement or inappropriately elevate perceptions of dangerousness.

Formulation

Once the caseload has been screened to identify the cases that meet the pathway criteria, there is a further filtering system to determine which cases are progressing on their sentence via standard offender management and which might benefit from specialist psychologically informed input to add value by facilitating progress and helping to manage risk. It is at this point that a decision is made about who enters the pathway and which services they will access. This can of course change over time and there are other opportunities to pick up missed cases or redirect to a more appropriate service. However, selecting appropriate individuals and understanding their risk and needs in order to plan a pathway of interventions are the defining steps of the OPD strategy [6, 35]. Prioritization is particularly important with a large cohort of offenders managed on scarce resources and requires a method that is both tailored to individual need and scalable to a widespread and highly morbid population. The OPD pathway selected formulation as the means to achieve this and this was probably an automatic choice based on its ubiquitous use in mental health.

There has been a surge of interest in forensic case formulation since 2012 [36–39]. This included an attempt to define the criteria of formulation and establish

Box 3.3 Definition of formulation

A statement of understanding about the whole person, explaining and connecting many aspects of their life experiences to the present point in time.

Source: data from Formulation Guidance for the Offender Personality Disorder Pathway, Unpublished (2014).

a standard [36], while the British Psychological Society set about a similar task in their Good Practice Guidelines [40]. The underlying drive was to improve quality and competence in formulation and measure it against the purpose for which it was being used. This was a constructive response to some views that the formulation process was esoteric, with mixed approaches in practice [40]. Up to this point, there had been few means of establishing the effectiveness of formulation, in terms of its grounding in psychological theory and its relationship to outcomes. It was against this backdrop that the OPD formulation approach was emerging.

Formulation has been defined by several authors, ranging from a more intricate description of 'a hypothesis about the causes, precipitants, and maintaining influences of a person's psychological, interpersonal and behavioral problems' [41] to 'a statement of understanding about the whole person, explaining and connecting many aspects of their life experiences to the present point in time' [40] (see Box 3.3). Formulation can feel at once both a simple and a complex task and it is the less well-defined ground between these two extremes that has provoked debate about the approach within the OPD pathway.

Introduction to formulation in the OPD pathway

The OPD strategy [6] placed formulation-led case management at the centre of the decision-making process for the pathway. Until this point, formulation had not been the routine approach for correctional services. Prison and probation would match offenders to large-scale manualized programmes according to risk, need, and responsivity [42,43] without recourse to individualized formulations. It could be argued that introducing formulation to offender management presumed an unmet need which had not been recognized—perhaps because in many cases a standard probation offence analysis was a sufficient level of understanding for less complex cases progressing well on their sentence.

However, ask a psychologist about the importance of formulation and it will be given unwavering support; it has been described as a 'lynchpin concept', the 'first principle', and the 'heart of evidence-based practice' [41]. It was perhaps understandable that OPD expected the criminal justice system to feel gratefully enlightened. Yet the introduction of formulation to the National Probation Service (NPS) has not been straightforward and there have been important lessons learned about necessary adaptations to the process and how to train professionals in its use. Questions remain about the utility of formulation in this context and its relationship to outcome. These issues are the focus of this section, following a brief overview of the literature.

Literature review

Although formulation might serve several purposes, its primary function is to help construct and implement interventions that lead to improved outcomes [41]. This relates to the core task of formulation in the OPD strategy [6]; to guide sentence planning to select the most appropriate interventions likely to reduce risk and improve psychological well-being. Beyond this, there are additional purposes that might have relevance for formulation in the criminal justice system. The British Psychological Society (BPS) [40] issued Good Practice Guidelines on the use of formulation and some of these seem clearly linked to objectives of the pathway (see Box 3.4).

The process of developing a formulation with a team can have a wider impact than on treatment planning alone. There are common problems encountered in the NPS where high caseloads and tight deadlines often lead to a paucity of information about service users and less thinking time to analyse risks and needs sufficiently to be able to plan ahead of time. This can lead to hurried crisis management, leaving the underlying issues that have driven problems unaddressed. This can have an impact on staff morale, result in team disagreements, and promote a culture of blame, which are likely to lead to risk-averse practice, less therapeutic risk taking, and reduced opportunities for positive change.

If the importance of formulation is accepted, the task of introducing formulation to professionals not accustomed to its use presents its own challenges. There is little research into the effectiveness of training in formulation; however, some results provide an indication of the issues at hand. First, there is only partial support for the extent to which formulation skills can be improved following a brief training. Three studies have indicated that clinicians have developed basic skills in formulation following training, but these improvements have not extended to more complex skills such as identifying underlying mechanisms [44]. Another study found clinicians moderately improved in fundamental elements of case formulation following a generic training, but there was significant space for further improvement [44]. In terms of the OPD pathway, we can conclude that brief training has only a partial impact, and more prolonged training or

Box 3.4 BPS guideline on uses of formulation

- Clarifying hypotheses and questions
- Noticing gaps in information about a service user
- Predicting responses to interventions
- Thinking about a lack of progress
- Helping the service user to feel contained
- Helping the therapist to feel contained
- Strengthening the therapeutic alliance
- Encouraging collaborative work with a service user
- Achieving a consistent team approach to interventions
- Generating new ways of thinking
- Dealing with core issues (not just crisis management)
- Reducing negative staff perceptions about service users
- Processing staff counter-transference reactions
- Helping staff to manage risk
- Minimizing disagreement and blame within teams
- Raising staff morale
- Conveying messages about hope for positive change

Source: data from British Psychological Society, Good Practice Guidelines on the use of Psychological Formulation, Copyright (2011), British Psychological Society.

practice-based tuition is indicated. These findings also raise the question of the extent of the formulation skills required for practitioners involved in the pathway—whether they need to develop expertise to identify complex internal psychological mechanisms or whether there is an acceptable level of competence which is adequate for the purposes required.

Second, there is evidence of a difference between novices and experts in the quality of formulations generated after both groups received the same training. On balance, experts develop formulations that are more elaborate, comprehensive, precise, complex, and more clearly matched to a treatment plan [44]. This has led to a call for a systematic coding system or checklist to enhance the evaluation of the quality of formulations [44]. More recently, there have been developments in this regard with at least two formulation quality checklists available

[40, 45]. However, it is unclear whether these checklists identify a threshold of adequate competence required for formulation in the pathway.

What is clear is that formulation continues to be highly valued and relied upon in mental health settings. There may be several reasons for this but not least that it has long been established as a core competency for mental health professionals [39] and so embedded in practice that perhaps its utility goes unquestioned. Despite this, there is little substantial evidence supporting a link between formulation and improved outcomes. One of the more persuasive studies involving depressed patients suggested formulation improved matching to more appropriate treatment plans which in turn led to improved outcomes for the patients [46]. However, other studies have suggested that standardized treatment programmes were as effective as formulation-driven treatment interventions [46]. The interventions in both conditions were suggested to be so powerful there was little room for improvement by formulation-driven treatment programmes. In the case of OPD pathway interventions, it is unlikely that standardized accredited programmes and personality disorder-specific interventions would have such a high treatment effect and so there would be more room to measure the impact of formulation-driven pathway planning. Currently, it remains an assumption that formulation in the pathway improves access to more appropriate treatments. On the strength of current evidence, it seems equivocal whether formulation directing to personality disorder-specific interventions would be any more effective than a standardized treatment plan for offenders. Further research into formulation and outcomes is desperately needed [40].

A final point from the literature relates to the different available approaches to formulation. These can be broadly divided into theoretically oriented formulations [41], problem-specific formulations [40], and generic atheoretical frameworks [41, 47]. A theoretical formulation is confined to the model it is based on and requires expertise in that field; problem-specific formulations are narrow in focus and usually limited to particular disorders. Neither seem suited to pathway formulations which require application to a variety of non-specific problems (e.g. an impasse in the pathway) and completion by a variety of professionals with different levels of expertise and knowledge of psychological theory. Generic frameworks appear to be the only appropriate option for community pathways formulations, which are co-constructed with offender managers and demand less expert knowledge. They have the advantage of being adaptable to numerous presenting problems (e.g. risk, clinical need, response to treatment), they do not constrain practitioners to one theoretical model, and they do not place undue demands on knowledge of psychological theory. Nevertheless, generic models such as the 'four P's' (predisposing, precipitating, perpetuating, and protective) [47] have their own limitations in that they provide little guidance about linking factors together and can result in a list of unrelated problems without an explanatory thread of personal meaning to the individual [40].

In considering appropriate models for formulation, it raises a related issue about matching formulation to task. In clinical settings, it is usual to adapt the level of formulation to the objective. For example, some formulations are comprehensive accounts of the individual and encompass the whole life story, whereas others might consist only of brief descriptions of maintaining cycles necessary to shift an individual [40]. Formulation-informed thinking is commonly used by psychologists as a means of communicating the meaning of behaviours to multi-disciplinary teams [40]. The selection of a partial or a full formulation might be influenced by resources of time and available information, efficiency (minimal formulation to meet the objective), and purpose. In transferring formulation to the OPD pathway, the same principle of adapting formulation to purpose should apply.

The LPP approach

The LPP approach to formulation evolved from early experiences of the pilot community pathways services in four boroughs of London between 2009 and 2011. It was designed to incorporate multiple functions, such as the process through which agencies come to a shared understanding of the risks and needs of an offender, to develop sentence planning including the selection and sequencing of interventions, the means by which teams can reflect on the impact of the work, to help resolve impasses, to inform and direct interventions within treatment services, and to improve insight via sharing the formulation with offenders. In recognition of variation in practice, we attempted to introduce a consistent approach to developing probation skills in formulation, to establish a model, and to agree a threshold for quality. The method followed recommendations from the literature and included psychoeducational training alongside practice-based learning, comprising a manualized training and half a year of monthly group case discussions focused on formulating offender manager cases. The model used was the Weerasekera [47] four P's approach which allowed psychological therapists the flexibility to incorporate theories in line with their expertise and did not require offender managers to have pre-existing knowledge of specific psychological approaches.

Despite the significant input, only half the offender managers improved their formulation skills significantly. Furthermore, the level of improvement remained well below a threshold of adequacy required by the quality checklist [45]. There may have been methodological reasons for the lack of improvement, such as the standard of the training and the consistent attendance of the offender managers in the training and group discussions. However, our over-riding impression from the data and our experience of running the project was of a limited buy-in to the process by offender managers and the inappropri-ateness of measuring quality against a standard expected of comprehensive formulations in clinical health settings [46]. Just as the level of detail should be adapted depending on the purpose of a formulation [40], so the threshold for quality should be adjusted accordingly. It seemed clear that the lack of in-vestment in the process from the offender managers was related to the per-ceived added value of formulation to their practice. Although some anecdotal accounts were positive, in attempting to introduce consistency by encouraging comprehensive formulations across the board, the level of detail often exceeded that which was necessary for the task. The formulations may have seemed too onerous and complex, without adding significant benefits.

The findings and experiences of this study informed a new stepped approach to formulation, designed to provide a method of matching the level of the for-mulation to the need [42]. This approach was latterly incorporated into the National Formulation Advisory Group and became the framework for for-mulation in the OPD pathway nationally. In brief, the stepped approach intro-duced three levels of formulation. A level 1 formulation describes a pattern of problem behaviours linked to an underlying psychological idea (see Box 3.5) and is used by offender managers for those progressing well on their sentence plan, or to help prison officers understand problematic behaviour. A level 2 formulation is more commonly used in less-intensive community or custody intervention settings (e.g. a Psychologically Informed Planned Environment (PIPE)) or where there is an impasse in the sentence plan. This level of formula-tion provides more of a narrative to explain the developmental history that led to the pattern of problem behaviours (see Box 3.6 in which the formulation re-garding Graham's behaviour is developed further). A level 3 formulation builds on the previous understanding by introducing psychological theory to support

Box 3.5 Level 1 formulation—a case example

Graham has two convictions for violence but self-reports many more inci-dents. Furthermore, the approved premises are complaining about his fre-quent loss of temper with staff. Triggers appear to include a sensitivity to other men who he feels treat him with disrespect—knocking over his drink, speaking rudely, or behaving in an off-hand manner in front of others. Graham insists that 'if you give an inch, they take the piss'.

Box 3.6 Level 2 formulation—a case example

Graham never knew his father; his mother could not cope with four children, and asked for Graham and his elder brother to be taken into care (but kept his younger brother). He was a badly behaved child, and foster care broke down a number of times, leading to long periods in a children's home. Graham insisted life in care was 'idyllic', he was the leader of the local gang, and he ran wild, involved in petty delinquency. He believed that the way to manage life was never to rely on others, and that all needs could be met through intimidation.

---

and explain how the developmental history led to the problematic behaviours. This highest level of formulation is usually developed by a psychological therapist and is recommended for use in secure treatment settings in hospital and prison and in intensive community interventions. This model is described in more detail in the Ministry of Justice publication 'Working with personality disordered offenders' [29].

The stepped approach allows enough flexibility to enable adaptation to need. This works well in group case discussions where the type of formulation has to be selected in the moment to fit the presenting problem. These can vary widely, including a stuck prisoner who has reached an impasse in their sentence, an analysis of an offence to understand motivation, a complex case bewildering the offender manager, an anxiety-provoking case evoking strong feelings in the team, or a better understanding of the risks and needs. The various purposes of formulation in the work with offender managers fit squarely with the BPS guidelines and incorporate many of their purposes listed earlier. The model has evolved to serve multiple functions in the pathways services which can potentially add value to the offender manager's routine practice.

The quality of formulations measured against a reasonable standard remains an issue. To date, the vast majority of the NPS caseload in London has been screened with a documented understanding of the case equivalent to at least a level 1 formulation. A significant number have level 2 or 3 formulations co-constructed between offender managers and pathway practitioners (psychological therapists or personality disorder probation officers). There is now an agreed national pathways audit tool for formulation [42] which has been piloted and will enable a threshold of quality to be established. This audit tool has been used to measure the effect of training on developing staff competence in formulation [49]. Shaw et al. [50] evaluated the impact of sharing formulations on the relationship between offender managers and service users, and on offender manager's clarity about case management priorities. Offender managers reported an improved quality of relationship, a stronger working alliance, and greater confidence in managing the case. Offenders reported trusting their offender managers more. The standard of formulation and its contribution to offender management is especially important where higher-risk cases are scrutinized more closely. In response to this, the LPP and London probation have developed an expectation that level 2 or 3 formulations should inform multi-agency public protection panel discussions.

Future directions

Moving forward, it will be interesting to see if the national audit tool will identify whether the greater number of level 1 formulations add meaningfully to an offender manager's practice. Formulation needs to be integrated into routine NPS practice to contribute significantly, and from our experience this means it will need to be accessible, of a reasonable standard of quality, and of added value. It is likely that only level 2 or 3 formulations with satisfy these criteria and we are now focusing on increasing their number.

A key aim of formulation in health settings is to come to a shared understanding of problems with the client [40]. The Community Pathways Service is mainly a consultation model involving little direct face-to-face work between personality disorder practitioners and offenders. This might be one reason why sharing formulations has not been a priority to date; however, this falls short of expectations and is an area that needs to be addressed. Co-working could be exploited for this purpose and there are other opportunities that could be explored further to encourage offender managers to share formulations with their clients.

An underpinning principle of the OPD pathway is a whole-systems approach, whereby continuity of care is promoted by a pathway of interventions across services and agencies, each building on the last [35]. This vision has not been fully realized, partly because formulations are not routinely shared between services. Within the LPP alone, formulations should continue to evolve and improve as they are shared between the Community Pathways Service, LPP prison services, and probation Approved Premises, to co-ordinate the approach and encourage continuity. This requires a culture shift within services, some of whom still act as stand-alone units providing a 'whole' treatment to the service user.

There is positive research to support the impact of the OPD pathway in London; higher-risk individuals are given more focus and progress further on the pathway [51], staff increase their awareness of risk with this group [52], and staff and offenders have a shared understanding of risk and desistance factors which echoes the literature [53]. These are all findings that could feasibly have been influenced by the use of formulation. However, none of the studies specifically evaluated whether formulation contributed to the improved outcomes. Formulation is now widespread in criminal justice settings, which offers more opportunities than ever before to find support for its use. We need to be clear whether formulation increases access to appropriate services by improving treatment planning and we need to establish whether formulation results in improved outcomes in terms of risk and psychosocial well-being. Support for this would require well-thought through research most likely carried out on a local level.

References

1. **Shaw J, Minoudis P, Craissati J.** A comparison of the Standardized Assessment of Personality—Abbreviated Scale and the offender assessment system personality disorder screen in a probation community sample. Journal of Forensic Psychiatry & Psychology. 2012 Apr 1;23(2):156–167.

2. **Pluck G, Brooker C, Blizard R, Moran P.** Personality disorder in a probation cohort: demographic, substance misuse, and forensic characteristics. Criminal Behaviour and Mental Health. 2015 Dec 1;25(5):403–415.

3. **Fazel S, Danesh J.** Serious mental disorder in 23,000 prisoners: a systematic review of 62 surveys. The Lancet. 2002 Feb 16;359(9306):545–550.

4. **Sirdifield C.** The prevalence of mental health disorders amongst offenders on probation: a literature review. Journal of Mental Health. 2012 Oct 1;21(5):485–498.

5. **Coid JW, Yang M, Ullrich S, Hickey N, Kahtan N, Freestone M.** Psychiatric diagnosis and differential risks of offending following discharge. International Journal of Law and Psychiatry. 2015 Feb 28;38:68–74.

6. **Joseph N, Benefield N.** A joint offender personality disorder pathway strategy: an outline summary. Criminal Behaviour and Mental Health. 2012 Jul 1;22(3):210–217.

7. **Ullrich S, Yang M, Coid J.** Dangerous and severe personality disorder: an investigation of the construct. International Journal of Law and Psychiatry. 2010 Apr 30;33(2):84–88.

8. **Grann M, Danesh J, Fazel S.** The association between psychiatric diagnosis and violent re-offending in adult offenders in the community. BMC Psychiatry. 2008 Nov 25;8(1):92.

9. **McMurran M, Huband N, Overton E.** Non-completion of personality disorder treatments: a systematic review of correlates, consequences, and interventions. Clinical Psychology Review. 2010 Apr 30;30(3):277–287.

10. **Trebilcock J, Weaver T.** Changing legal characteristics of dangerous and severe personality disorder (DSPD) patients and prisoners. Journal of Forensic Psychiatry & Psychology. 2012 Apr 1;23(2):237–243.

11. **Loranger AW.** Are current self-report and interview measures adequate for epidemiological studies of personality disorders? Journal of Personality Disorders. 1992 Dec 1;6(4):313.

12. **Blackburn R, Fawcett D.** The antisocial personality questionnaire: an inventory for assessing personality deviation in offender populations. European Journal of Psychological Assessment. 1999;15(1):14.

13. **Moran P, Leese M, Lee T, Walters P, Thornicroft G, Mann A.** Standardized Assessment of Personality—Abbreviated Scale (SAPAS): preliminary validation of a brief screen for personality disorder. British Journal of Psychiatry. 2003 Sep 1;**183**(3):228–232.

14. **Furnham A, Milner R, Akhtar R, De Fruyt F.** A review of the measures designed to assess DSM-5 personality disorders. Psychology. 2014 Sep 30;5(14):1646.

15. **Tew J, Harkins L, Dixon L.** Assessing the reliability and validity of the Self-Report Psychopathy Scales in a UK offender population. Journal of Forensic Psychiatry & Psychology. 2015 Mar 4;**26**(2):166–184.

16. **Guy LS, Poythress NG, Douglas KS, Skeem JL, Edens JF.** Correspondence between self-report and interview-based assessments of antisocial personality disorder. Psychological Assessment. 2008 Mar;**20**(1):47.

17. **Pluck G, Brooker C, Blizard R, Moran P.** Personality disorder in a probation cohort: demographic, substance misuse and forensic characteristics. Criminal Behaviour and Mental Health. 2015 Dec 1;**25**(5):403–415.

18. **Howard P, Moore R.** Measuring changes in risk and need over time using OASys. London: Ministry of Justice. 2009.

19. **Craissati J, Webb L, Keen S.** The relationship between developmental variables, personality disorder, and risk in sex offenders. Sexual Abuse: A Journal of Research and Treatment. 2008 Jun 1;**20**(2):119–138.

20. **Bui L, Ullrich S, Coid JW.** Screening for mental disorder using the UK national offender assessment system. Journal of Forensic Psychiatry & Psychology. 2016 Nov 1;**27**(6):786–801.

21. **Shaw J, Edelmann R.** Predictors of engagement, understanding and dropout from a community based cognitive skills programme. (Manuscript submitted for publication.)

22. **Yu R, Geddes JR, Fazel S.** Personality disorders, violence, and antisocial behavior: a systematic review and meta-regression analysis. Journal of Personality Disorders. 2012 Oct 1;**26**(5):775.

23. **McMurran M, Howard R (Eds.).** Personality, personality disorder and violence: an evidence based approach. Chichester: John Wiley & Sons; 2009.

24. **Nestor PG.** Mental disorder and violence: personality dimensions and clinical features. American Journal of Psychiatry. 2002 Dec;**159**(12):1973–1978.

25. **Minoudis P, Shaw J, Bannerman A, Craissati J.** Identifying personality disturbance in a London probation sample. Probation Journal. 2012 Mar 1;**59**(1):23–38.

26. **Morton S.** Can OASys deliver consistent assessments of offenders? Results from the inter-rater reliability study. Research Summary 1(09). London: Ministry of Justice; 2009.

27. **González RA, Kallis C, Ullrich S, Barnicot K, Keers R, Coid JW.** Childhood maltreatment and violence: mediation through psychiatric morbidity. Child Abuse & Neglect. 2016 Feb 29;**52**:70–84.

28. **London Pathways Partnership.** Case identification audit. Unpublished report. London Pathways Partnership; 2015.

29. **Craissati J, Joseph N, Skett S (Eds.).** Working with personality disordered offenders: a practitioner's guide. London: Ministry of Justice; 2015.

30. **NHS England Commissioning Support Unit.** High level analysis of OPD data returns. Unpublished report. NHS England Commissioning Support Unit; 2015.

31. Nichols F, Dunster C, Beckley K. Identifying personality disturbance in the Lincolnshire personality disorder pathway: how do offenders compare to the London pilot? Probation Journal. 2016 Mar 1;**63**(1):41–53.

32. Craissati J, Sindall O. Serious further offences: an exploration of risk and typologies. Probation Journal. 2009 Mar 1;**56**(1):9–27.

33. Ndegwa D. Personality disorder in African and African-Caribbean people in the UK. London: Department of Health.

34. Cattell J, Minoudis P, Shaw J. An evaluation of the London Pathways Partnership services for offenders with personality disorder. Paper presented at the British and Irish Group for the Study of Personality Disorders (BIGSPD), 15 March 2016, Isle of Man.

35. Minoudis P, Shaw J, Craissati J. The London Pathways project: evaluating the effectiveness of a consultation model for personality disordered offenders. Criminal Behaviour and Mental Health. 2012 Jul 1;**22**(3):218–232.

36. Hart S, Sturmey P, Logan C, McMurran M. Forensic case formulation. International Journal of Forensic Mental Health. 2011 Apr 1;**10**(2):118–126.

37. McMurran M, Taylor PJ. Case formulation with offenders: what, who, where, when, why and how? Criminal Behaviour and Mental Health. 2013 Oct 1;**23**(4):227–229.

38. Völlm B. Case formulation in personality disordered offenders—a Delphi survey of professionals. Criminal Behaviour and Mental Health. 2014 Feb 1;**24**(1):60–80.

39. Sturmey P, McMurran M (Eds.). Forensic case formulation. London: John Wiley & Sons; 2011.

40. British Psychological Society. Good practice guidelines on the use of psychological formulation. Leicester: The British Psychological Society; 2011.

41. Eells TD, Lombart KG. Theoretical and evidence-based approaches to case formulation. Forensic Case Formulation. 2011 Sep 22:1–32.

42. Ministry of Justice. Working with personality disordered offenders: a practitioner's guide. Chapter 3: Formulation. London: Ministry of Justice. 2017, pp. 37–47.

43. Bonta J, Andrews DA. Risk–need–responsivity model for offender assessment and rehabilitation. Rehabilitation. 2007;**6**:1–22.

44. Mumma GH. Current issues in case formulation. Forensic Case Formulation. 2011 Sep 22:33–60.

45. McMurran M, Logan C, Hart S. Case formulation quality checklist. Nottingham: Institute of Mental Health; 2012.

46. Ghaderi A. Does case formulation make a difference to treatment outcome? Forensic Case Formulation. 2011 Sep 22:61–79.

47. Weerasekera P. Multiperspective case formulation: a step towards treatment integration. Malabar, FL: Krieger Publishing Company; 1996.

48. Minoudis P, Craissati J, Shaw J, McMurran M, Freestone M, Chuan SJ, Leonard A. An evaluation of case formulation training and consultation with probation officers. Criminal Behaviour and Mental Health. 2013 Oct 1;**23**(4):252–262.

49. Ramsden J, Lowton M, Joyes E. The impact of case formulation focussed consultation on criminal justice staff and their attitudes to work with personality disorder. Mental Health Review Journal. 2014 Jun 3;**19**(2):124–130.

50. **Shaw J, Higgins C, Quartey C.** The impact of collaborative case formulation with high risk offenders with personality disorder. Journal of Forensic Psychiatry & Psychology. **28**:777–789.

51. **Jolliffe D, Cattell J, Raza A, Minoudis P.** Factors associated with progression in the London Pathway Project. Criminal Behaviour and Mental Health. 2017;**27**(3):222–237.

52. **Jolliffe D, Cattell J, Raza A, Minoudis P.** Evaluating the impact of the London Pathway Project. Criminal Behaviour and Mental Health. 2017;**27**(3):238–253.

53. **McMurran M, Delight S.** Processes of change in an offender personality disorder pathway prison progression unit. Criminal Behaviour and Mental Health. 2017;**27**(3):254–264.

Chapter 4

Intervening in the community

Jackie Craissati and Rob Halsey

Introduction

With the new OPD pathway strategy, there has been a clear shift to focusing on the community as central to the pathway. Offender managers, located in local offices throughout England and Wales, are the case managers for all offenders, from the point of conviction through custody and back into society when released on licence. In principle and, more often than not, in practice, they drive the sentence plan and push for progression where possible. Of the 20,000 or so high-risk offenders with pervasive psychological problems, half to two-thirds are estimated to be in the community at any one time, and it is stating the obvious to point out that this is where the risk to the public is most acute. Furthermore, it is only when back in the community that we can really know whether our interventions have worked, in terms of the ultimate test of success—leading an offence-free life.

This chapter briefly reviews the relevant literature for community interventions, both therapy and management approaches, and considers the options for intervention that are in line with the ethos of the community approach. It details the core tasks of the strategy—identification, formulation, consultation, and training—and reviews progress to date.

What we currently know

Treatment interventions

There is a modest but growing literature evaluating the outcome of psychological interventions for both criminal justice targets and personality disorder. However, the research studies in these areas are limited by their relatively weak design and methodology; samples tend to be biased; there are limited control groups; and outcomes are variably assessed by self-report questionnaires, therapist observations, health outcomes, or reoffending. Thus, relying on the results of individual studies is uncertain, but even drawing conclusions from larger reviews of the literature remains tentative.

Probably the most helpful reports for the interested reader are as detailed in Box 4.1.

The key findings from research are summarized below. The focus has been restricted to community studies only, and an attempt has been made to separate out interventions designed to target personality (and associated traits) as compared to those targeting problem behaviours (such as offending or substance misuse), although there are inevitably overlaps, most notably in the case of anti-social personality disorder (ASPD).

Box 4.1 Evidence-based interventions for personality disordered offenders—further reading

NICE guidelines for individuals with ASPD and BPD (2013, https://www.nice. org.uk/guidance)

The National Institute for Health and Care Excellence provides health guidance on the assessment, treatment, and management of personality disorder, drawing on good-quality research evidence, and their criteria and conclusions are rather broader than those of Cochrane (see below).

Transforming rehabilitation: a summary of evidence on reducing reoffending (Ministry of Justice Analytical Series, 2013, https://www.gov.uk/government/ uploads/system/uploads/attachment_data/file/243718/evidence-reduce-reof-fending.pdf)

This review lays out the strength of the current evidence base for a range of interventions addressing common dynamic risk factors in offenders, and factors related to desistance.

Cochrane Reviews for psychological interventions for ASPD (2010) and BPD (2012); for adults who have sexually offended (2012); and for men who have physically abused their partners (2011) (http://www.cochrane. org/evidence)

Cochrane Reviews offer a review and analysis of high-quality studies—usually randomized control trials—on a range of topics.

Craig, Dixon, and Gannon (Eds.). What works in offender rehabilitation: an evidence-based approach to assessment and treatment. Chichester: Wiley-Blackwell; 2013

This edited volume summarizes the evidence base for a range of interventions in relevant settings, for a diverse range of offence-related behaviours.

Borderline personality disorder (BPD) has been most frequently studied in the community, and the most commonly compared therapies have included dialectical behaviour therapy (DBT), mentalization-based therapy (MBT), transference-focused therapy (TFP), and schema-focused therapy (SFT). Standard DBT and MBT offer a combination of individual and group therapy; TFP and SFT are more flexible in their delivery, often relying on individual work alone. DBT—the most widely studied of the therapies—has also established that the skills training component is the most important element for effecting sustained therapeutic change [1]; that is, DBT is most effective at reducing the frequency of behavioural problems associated with impulsivity (but less effective at improving mood states or interpersonal functioning). All four therapies are equally able to demonstrate significantly greater effectiveness than standard care or non-expert therapies, but the evidence to support their superiority over the other expert therapies is less robust.

ASPD has been much less widely studied, and meta-analytic approaches have not been able to identify robust and sustained outcomes, in terms of re-offending, aggression, or social functioning. Interestingly, the most promising results have come from studies looking at ASPD and substance misuse, where reduction in substance use was measured following contingency management (where progress in not using substances is rewarded) and cognitive behavioural interventions. The one randomized control trial in the community, for people with ASPD [2], found that a cognitive behavioural intervention was a relatively expensive option compared to treatment as usual, with no significant effect in reducing anger or aggression. These findings, perhaps, exemplify the challenge in demonstrating a functional link between the personality type and the offending behaviour, as interventions have been demonstrably more successful with the latter than the former.

The evidence in relation to a reduction in offending behaviour is a little more promising, although still modest. The most common community intervention of relevance is thinking skills. Although programme names and content change, these interventions all target poor decision making, impulsive behaviour, and flawed social problem-solving skills. These traits are likely to overlap with antisocial traits, although the programmes do not specify personality disorder as an inclusion criteria. Hollin et al. [3] compared over 2,000 offenders on a probation order and participating in a cognitive skills group, with a similar-sized control group, and found that programme completion was associated with a significantly lower reconviction rate. The caveat to this encouraging finding is that only 30% of the sample completed the programme, and there is the possibility—albeit speculative—that those with more marked antisocial traits were more likely to be the participants that dropped out (and reoffended at a higher rate).

The issue of treatment drop-out—not to be confused with treatment refusal—is of particular salience in relation to personality disordered offenders. Not only are the variables associated with increased likelihood of drop-out strongly linked to personality disorder traits [4], but also those who drop out are generally about twice as likely to reoffend sexually or violently as compared to a matched control group [5]. This becomes particularly salient in the community, when chaotic lifestyles and impulsive decision making raises the likelihood of individuals failing to complete programmes. Although treatment attrition is a disadvantage of community treatment delivery, this needs to be balanced against the advantages—most notably, the slightly superior treatment effect found in community interventions [6]. Effect sizes—found in meta-analytic studies to be moderate (around 25%) rather than large—can also be improved when interventions attend to the risk–needs–responsivity principles (to around 50% less likelihood of reoffending [7]). That is, intervening with higher-risk offenders—who display a greater frequency of undesirable behaviours—with greater dosage of therapy addressing a greater range of behaviours, and minimizing the drop-out rate, yields the optimum results.

Interventions for other types of personality disorder have rarely been evaluated robustly; and indeed, Cochrane Review groups have withdrawn its protocols for interventions for narcissistic and for avoidant personality disorder due to difficulties in identifying potentially suitable studies. There are a few examples of studies with a wider group of personality disordered individuals: a large multi-centred randomized control trial of schema therapy in the Netherlands included a full range of personality types. This study established the superiority of SFT as compared to treatment as usual or clarification-oriented psychotherapy, as well as the superiority of exercise-based schema therapy training to lecture-based training. Although less methodologically robust, Craissati and Blundell [8] published a range of research results on the characteristics and treatment outcomes of a programme for personality disordered sex offenders, reporting on a range of personality types, with significant treatment effects for high-risk sex offenders.

Summarizing briefly:

- There is some evidence to suggest that psychological interventions that are specifically designed for individuals with personality disorder do make a unique contribution to positive outcomes.

- Outcomes may actually be more closely related to clear and coherent models of care and treatment protocols than to the specific content of various therapies; there is little evidence for the superiority of one therapy over another.

◆ Targeting behaviours that are associated with personality disorder (self-harm, substance misuse, general offending) may also lead to positive outcomes, although it is important to pay particular attention to those who are likely to drop out of treatment.

Management approaches

There is very little published regarding the evaluation of innovative approaches to managing personality disordered offenders, as opposed to delivering treatment interventions. There is a small literature on the role that personality disorder plays in increasing the complexity of the work within mainstream community mental health approaches [9] and published reviews on more intensive community management approaches for offenders (including thematic probation inspection reports for persistent and prolific offender schemes [10]). General psychiatric management (or what Bateman variously describes as structured clinical management, or good clinical care [11]) has been shown to be as effective as specialist treatments in the management of some individuals with BPD. However, these so-called mainstream community care approaches are in fact enhanced approaches to management, which include structured protocols with the following features:

◆ A manualized structure to support the clinician

◆ Encouragement of increased activity and self-agency for the patients

◆ A focus on emotional processing, creating robust connections between acts and feeling

◆ Including a model of pathology which is carefully explained to patients

◆ Encouraging an active clinician stance, including an explicit intention to validate and to generate a strong therapeutic alliance.

In terms of criminal justice approaches, the development of Multi-Agency Public Protection Arrangements (MAPPA) is probably the most significant development in the community management of offenders in recent years. MAPPA was introduced in England and Wales in 2001 under the Criminal Justice and Court Services Act (2000, sections 67 and 68) to facilitate the sharing of information amongst agencies to improve public protection. Police, probation and prison services form the responsible authority with a statutory duty to ensure that the risks posed by specified sexual and violent offenders are assessed and managed appropriately, and other agencies—such as health, youth justice, and the local authority—have a 'duty to co-operate' (Criminal Justice Act, 2003, section 325 [3]). MAPPA is not a stand-alone integrated management team but represents innovative partnership working (see below) which appears to be making a contribution to reducing sexual and violent reconviction rates [12]. The vast majority of high-risk or high-harm offenders with personality disorder will be subject to MAPPA once out in the community, and subject to participating agency decisions regarding community access and third-party disclosure.

The Parole Board for England and Wales was established in 1968 and is an 'arms-length' court-like body, funded by but independent of the Ministry of Justice for England and Wales. The Parole Board is responsible for release decisions for all prisoners who are subject to indeterminate prison sentences (including life sentences and sentences for public protection), a significant proportion of whom will fall within the remit of the OPD pathway. Released on life licence, such offenders will be subject to indefinite supervision by the probation service. Outcomes for Parole Board decisions tend to be fairly stable and good, with released indeterminate-sentenced prisoners demonstrating a reoffending rate (for sexual and violent crime over four years on licence in the community) averaging 3% [13]. Although indeterminate sentences were never conceptualized on the basis of clinical factors, the demonstrable success of the system does chime with key constructs now explicit within the OPD pathway: that is, the sentence integrates punishment (the tariff element of the sentence which is 'done to' the prisoner) with the potential for rehabilitation for which the prisoner must take active responsibility if he/she is to convince the Parole Board of meaningful change.

The most creative innovations in recent years have arguably emerged from voluntary sector organizations; for example, the expansion of Circles of Support and Accountability (COSA). These have spread from delivery in small areas in rural North America to an established international presence, including increasing availability in the UK. Circles were first developed in Canada in the mid-1990s based on the principles of restorative justice [14]. They began as an informal community response to fears evoked by the release of high-risk child sex offenders into the community, where individuals, mainly of the Mennonite faith, formed small groups or 'circles' around the released offenders. COSA aims to promote community integration of offenders by helping them develop and maintain engagement in positive activities and supportive relationships within the community. There are currently ten COSA projects in England and Wales. A descriptive study of a well-established UK COSA, covering an eight-year period, reported one sexual reconviction among the sixty core members reviewed [15]. In addition, 70% of the sample attributed improvements in well-being to the support they received from their 'circle'. In a series of controlled studies based in Canada, it was found that involvement in a 'circle' significantly reduces reconviction rates amongst those assessed as most likely to reoffend sexually. A review [16] suggests that COSA not only reduces reoffending rates in high-risk sexual offenders but also promotes prosocial attitudes and activities.

Although COSA has restricted their remit to child sex offenders, some community projects for high-risk personality disordered offenders have been heavily influenced by the model and have adapted it to work with those with adult victims and those with histories of physical violence. A preliminary mixed method evaluation of one example—Sova Support Link—demonstrated high levels of service user and referrer satisfaction with the service, high levels of engagement, and modest improvements in psychosocial functioning. This service was compared to a resettlement project with an identical ethos (the former delivering the service with volunteers and the latter with paid social care staff) in terms of a service user perspective and found that there were similar levels of satisfaction and community integration with both models [17].

A related development—particularly widespread in the US but also emerging in the UK—are community notification approaches, specifically in relation to child sexual abusers. These include a variety of methods to provide neighbourhoods and concerned members of the public with varying amounts of information regarding possible sex offenders in their area or known to them [18]. Preliminary evaluations of these projects suggest that although the schemes are popular with the general public, there is no evidence that reoffending risk is reduced as a result of these approaches. A comparable scheme in relation to domestic violence offenders was launched in England and Wales in 2014 following a fourteen-month pilot [19]. Of 386 requests, 29% resulted in a disclosure. Again, those involved in the pilot were positive, but as yet there has been no published evidence regarding its effectiveness as a management approach.

Options available

Before considering the range of intervention models available, it is important to pay attention to the context in which services are to be delivered. The availability of suitable resources—whether this be physical space or staffing—may restrict options. For example, difficulties with the recruitment and retention of a skilled workforce pose significant obstacles to the delivery of a consistent and high-quality service; the appetite of the organizations involved (notably health) to engage with work with personality disordered offenders may vary hugely. There may also be organizational imperatives that dictate whether or not a service should target particular problem groups of offenders, or particular geographical locations; concerns regarding equal access and comprehensive delivery may necessitate the delivery of a leaner intervention with the deployment of limited staffing resources.

The challenges posed by service delivery in a largely rural area, as compared to delivery in a densely populated urban area, include the availability of a suitable client group (perhaps sharing the necessary characteristics for a particular intervention) and the problems of excessive travel requirements for both staff and offenders. These difficulties are not insurmountable, but more creativity in delivery may be required in rural areas, perhaps with greater emphasis on the co-ordination of appointments, or, for example, longer duration of interventions over a shorter period of time with greater use of telephone contact and messaging support.

Decisions regarding interventions are also likely to be influenced by the availability of complementary or support services. This can be a positive feature; for example, the presence of a non-forensic personality disorder service can be supported to expand their remit to include personality disordered offenders, thereby deploying limited resources efficiently. Conversely, problems with accessing meaningful activity and suitable housing can destabilize or impair the impact of any bespoke intervention for personality disordered offenders, where the benefits of any intervention are undermined by lifestyle instability and offenders struggling with preoccupied feelings of grievance and hopelessness. In urban areas, this is often exacerbated by heightened proximity to antisocial peers, a significant risk factor for those with antisocial traits.

The following four models for designing delivery of services therefore need to be weighed up in the light of contextual factors. The models are summarized in Table 4.1.

Stand-alone treatment approach

The option of stand-alone treatment is familiar to health services and involves the delivery of an evidence-based community treatment programme, receiving referrals from the CJS. As detailed in the section on published evaluations ('Treatment interventions'), examples include SFT, DBT, and MBT services. There are advantages to this model, not least the availability of a modest but positive evidence base in relation to non-forensic community service outcomes, and the ability of health to provide skilled and confident practitioners. Model integrity is easier to monitor and maintain, and the lines of responsibility are clear. A referral is logged onto the health 'patient information system' which is associated with clear quality standards for the health intervention.

However, there are significant disadvantages to a stand-alone treatment approach, and this largely relates to the gatekeeping with which it is inevitably

Table 4.1 Summary of delivery options: Health and criminal justice system (CJS) working together

Option	Advantages	Disadvantages
a. **Stand-alone treatment approach** Health delivers an evidence-based community treatment programme, receiving referrals from the CJS	◆ There is an evidence base for specific treatments, for which health is trained and competent to deliver ◆ The impact on the clients who complete the programme may be strong. The integrity of the model is easier to maintain, as is delivery ◆ Health assumes responsibility for the client for the duration of treatment	◆ There is a risk of treatment criteria resulting in excessive gatekeeping and exclusion of the most challenging clients. Fewer clients receive the service, which is expensive to deliver ◆ Health is likely to lack influence over CJS interventions, while assuming high levels of responsibility and risk to the organization
b. **Partnership working** Health delivers interventions in parallel with CJS interventions, with co-ordination and exchange of information	◆ The delivery of interventions by health are enhanced by close working with the CJS, leading to some sharing of expertise and responsibility for outcomes ◆ Costs may be lowered as a result and the impact may be improved in terms of outcomes	◆ Partnerships may result in fragmentation and splitting, mirroring client difficulties. There is a risk of blurring of boundaries and potential confusion regarding responsibilities ◆ Inefficiencies may occur with duplication of approaches ◆ There may be conflict between organizational policies and procedures
c. **Indirect support** Health delivers consultation and training to CJS staff, who in turn deliver the intervention	◆ There is greater clarity of roles and responsibilities, with health adopting the 'expert' role ◆ Delivery is cost effective, with potential for generalization of learning for CJS staff, to enable improved management of a wide range of clients	◆ The availability of 'experts' may inadvertently reduce feelings of competence in the CJS, with increased dependency on health for knowledge ◆ The impact may be reduced in terms of lack of influence on organizational practice

(continued)

Table 4.1 Continued

Option	Advantages	Disadvantages
d. **Integrated delivery** Health and the CJS work in new ways together to offer new, shared interventions	◆ Working with new teams and models of intervention can promote innovation and new ways of programme delivery. There are opportunities for motivating staff and improving impact on outcomes ◆ Risk is fully shared, and roles and responsibilities become more generic and equal between agencies	◆ Integrated working is difficult to embed within large organizations, with resistance to changing policies and procedures for special projects, and misunderstanding the model ◆ This may raise risk issues when difficulties occur. Roles and responsibilities may be unclear

associated. The attrition rate from referral to treatment acceptance to treatment completion tends to be high in non-forensic treatment programmes, and extremely high (around 90%—personal communication, OPD pathway network meeting) in forensic programmes. In the effort to maintain treatment effectiveness, the majority of offenders referred—those who are most challenging on account of their ambivalent motivation, lack of reflective capacity, chaotic lifestyles, and problems with impulsivity—are unlikely to benefit from the service. These barriers to entry—most particularly the stigma associated with diagnosis, mental health, and hospital services—are particularly striking for young adult offenders and those from a black and minority ethnic background, who are less likely to consider talking therapy, with its white middle-class bias, as relevant to them. The end result risks alienating the CJS referrers, while deploying a relatively expensive resource for a small number of the more manageable offenders. In attempting to reduce the barriers to entry, health is likely to be highly anxious about the risk implications of delivering a stand-alone service to more challenging offenders who may well reoffend (or otherwise put pressure on wider health resources), with associated reputational risks for the service.

Partnership working

Partnership working, as defined here, involves the delivery of parallel services (health and CJS) but with a more formalized relationship (protocols, service-level agreements, and/or contracts), including co-ordination and the exchange of information between services. Partnership models are discussed more fully in Chapter 7. Partnership working is often a feature of case management (and sentence planning) approaches which organize the delivery of complementary contracted services to intervene with various aspects of the offender's presenting difficulties. MAPPA (described in the section 'Management approaches') could also be considered as a partnership model, which combines shared decision making around risk with parallel service delivery; this is also true of many court diversion or police liaison schemes. This approach has significant advantages, in terms of each agency's ability to deliver within their mainstream approach, thereby keeping additional costs to a minimum; it plays to each agency's strengths, and where roles and responsibilities are delineated but shared [20] there are opportunities for improving the impact of collective interventions. For health, this offers the additional advantage of risk sharing, which reduces— but does not altogether eliminate—anxieties regarding organizational reputation; however, information exchange is not always straightforward, as there are entirely separate and potentially different standards in relation to professional codes of conduct, confidentiality, and disclosure.

The disadvantages of parallel partnerships largely relate to the potential for fragmentation and splitting between agencies that mirror the presenting problems of the offender. This is particularly so for those with personality disorder, who present primarily with relational difficulties, where difficulties can emerge at the practitioner level as well as the organizational level. This is beautifully described by Davies [21]:

> 'The view is taken that professionals who deal with offenders are not free agents but potential actors who have been assigned roles in the individual offender's own re-enactment of their internal world drama. The professionals have the choice not to perform but they can only make this choice when they have a good idea of what the role is they are trying to avoid. Until they can work this out they are likely to be drawn into the play, unwittingly and therefore not unwillingly. Because of the latter, if the pressure to play is not anticipated then the professional will believe he is in a role of his choosing. Unfortunately, initially, only a preview of the plot is available in the somewhat cryptic form of the offence .... It is also important to comment that it is not only the offender's internal drama that professionals are called upon to enact but also those more explicit scripts of their own organizations and central government. They will also be under pressure from themselves to re-enact their own dramas.'

Indirect support

Indirect support is a familiar model to psychological therapists, with the delivery of indirect interventions to CJS staff—namely consultation and training—which in turn inform the delivery of CJS interventions for personality disordered offenders. There is a published literature on consultation models and theoretical principles, although nothing robust that measures its effectiveness in terms of outcomes for offenders. The evaluation literature on training of CJS staff is a little more developed (see Chapter 2), with demonstrable effectiveness in promoting increased confidence and competence in the workforce. There are considerable advantages to this model in terms of cost effectiveness, the intervention having the potential to be delivered to a number of staff in a group setting and to have a generalizable impact on effectiveness; but also in terms of the organizational risk to health services of working with this complex offender group, as there is no 'ownership' of the offender with associated responsibility for his/her behaviour. This is an 'expert' model which carries both advantages and disadvantages: it can have a significant positive impact on the morale and confidence of CJS practitioners, who feel supported and contained by the expertise of the consultant, but it is important not to engender dependence on the consultant, which inadvertently undermines the expertise of the CJS practitioner. What the consultant or trainer gains in terms of risk avoidance may need to be balanced against the loss of control that is associated with indirect working; that is, the impact of the intervention may be lost 'in translation'.

Integrated delivery

Prior to the inception of the OPD strategy, there were few, if any, examples of truly integrated working between health and the CJS. Integrated delivery requires new models and ways of working which break down traditional roles and responsibilities and organizational procedures, and which can therefore be difficult to embed, and are vulnerable to being misunderstood by or isolated from other elements of the participating organizations. They are persistently susceptible to the tendency to drift back into familiar ways of working which undermine the integrated model. Organizations are peculiarly resistant to new policies and procedures that are service specific, and therefore an agreement to operate an integrated service might not be accompanied by an agreement to develop shared policies and procedures around risk, care planning, decision making, and confidentiality. However, a fully integrated service does bring huge possibilities for innovation, and often attracts motivated and skilled staff who develop ownership of the service model and its delivery.

How we chose our approach

The approach adopted by the London Pathways Partnership (LPP) consortium was essentially pragmatic and, instead of deciding upon one particular model and rejecting all others (and thereby losing the advantages inherent in each), an attempt was made to extract the positive aspects from each of the models.

The key community challenge was to deploy relatively scarce resources across twenty three delivery areas within London, and in doing so, identify the right offenders from the 50,000 on the London probation caseload, intervene or enhance sentence planning where necessary, and train almost 2,000 staff.

Delivery areas, in the London context, refer to the boroughs, of which there are thirty two, around which probation services are organized (referred to as local delivery units (LDUs)); outside London, delivery units may refer to a whole county or to part of a county. The task reduced somewhat following the splitting off of lower-risk offenders to the privately owned Community Rehabilitation Companies (CRC), but remained onerous. The CRCs were set up in 2013, as part of the government's Transforming Rehabilitation (TR) strategy in England and Wales, in order to reform the ways in which offenders are managed. The context for delivery was an ever-changing staff group with variable experience, working with a complex range of offenders—including a high level of gang and extremist offenders, and comorbid substance misuse offenders—against a wider social environment of very significant problems, including limited access to housing and employment opportunities and soaring daily living expenses.

Theoretical model

Theoretically, we were clear that criminological work around desistance, coupled with attachment theory, provided our overarching approach to a model of care (see Chapter 1 for a more detailed explanation of these models). These models influenced our approach to formulation and treatment, and our choice of third-sector (charity) partners. It was important to us that our approach to working with personality disordered offenders was hopeful and positive in orientation, focused on progression, and with attention paid to the interpersonal features of the disorder which complicate perceptions of risk and can often induce impasse for the offender and burnout for the probation officer.

Operational model

What distinguished the implementation of the OPD pathway from any previous venture was the community focus, coupled with an intention to move away from a bespoke expert delivery. It was therefore crucial that the operational delivery ensured that an offender would receive equal access to available services, regardless of where he/she resided. Staffing is described in more detail in Chapter 2. Suffice to say, every LDU had access to a half-time personality disorder probation officer (PDPO) who worked alongside a psychologist therapist (available for one day a week per LDU and for half a day a week for each probation hostel). This core service was supplemented—across London—by a specialist MBT programme for violent antisocial offenders and a specialist sex offender programme for personality disordered sex offenders. Finally, our third-sector partners provided access to meaningful relationships with non-professional others and valued work roles, which enhanced offender perceptions of their developing sense of themselves as hopeful members of the community.

In brief—and somewhat oversimplified—the LPP consortium aspired to offer an accessible and value-added service to all probation staff in London that would enable them to deliver a better targeted and more thoughtful service to all high-risk offenders with pervasive psychological difficulties. In doing so, this would enable the workforce to develop resilience in the face of challenging interpersonal dynamics; and achieve better outcomes for the offender in terms of maximizing opportunities for them to lead offence-free lives in the community.

Core tasks

We adopted an integrated approach to partnership for all the core tasks, which were delivered from within probation offices and hostels. The core tasks included:

+ Ensuring that all probation officers attended training which developed their understanding of personality disorder and their skills in managing these more challenging offenders (see Chapter 2 on staff training and selection)

+ The appropriate identification of offenders with traits likely to meet diagnostic criteria for personality disorder, albeit not requiring the diagnosis (see Chapter 3 for more detail)

+ Arriving at a more psychologically informed understanding of their difficulties (see Chapter 3 for formulation), in collaboration with the probation officer

+ Occasionally working briefly with the probation officer and the offender together, in order to resolve a dilemma (joint case work).

Fig. 4.1 outlines the approach and the approximate numbers involved for London. This filtering system was based on the premise that the core service aimed to support the offender manager in delivery in the most efficient manner possible; that is, where the sentence plan was in hand and progressing well, there was no need to intervene, even if the offender met OPD pathway criteria.

Although the exact figures are in flux, Fig. 4.1 provides a reasonable snapshot of activity within the OPD pathway in London in 2016. The proportion of offenders screened into the pathway is around one-third of the total caseload of London probation, of whom around 40% are in prison at any one time, and the remainder in the community. For many of those screened in, the probation conceptualization of the offence, the risk, and the required sentence plan was good, and the offenders were progressing according to plan. However, on the basis of

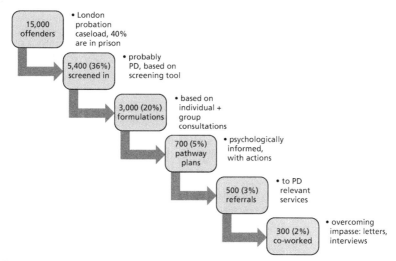

Fig. 4.1 Schematic view of the community operational delivery

individual and group consultations with the offender managers (OM), around 3,000 formulations have been completed and written up, their purpose being to review and amend the sentence plan in light of a more psychologically informed conceptualization of the offender's behaviour or difficulties in progression. For those already in the community, formulations have been important in trying to support staff in stabilizing chaotic presentations or challenging behaviour. For a significant minority of offenders, OPD pathway staff made recommendations for referral to specific services, in order to try to overcome impasse or access potentially helpful interventions.

Although many aspects of the core tasks are covered in detail in other chapters, it is worth pausing here to discuss in a little more detail the role of consultation and our approach to co-working.

Consultation is a core skill for many practitioners, but does raise anxieties for some in terms of understanding the scope of their professional and agency responsibility. We therefore found it helpful to delineate exactly what we were referring to as consultation, the standard expected and associated risks, as well as the focus. The following is an extract from our guidance:

'For the purposes of the OPD pathway, consultation normally refers to the verbal interaction or discussion between a pathway practitioner (either a psychological therapist or a PD probation officer) and an offender manager (OM), in relation to a particular offender. Consultation may encompass advice-giving and signposting. This may take place on a one to one basis, or in a group format. It is the responsibility of the consultee to provide information that is as accurate and relevant as possible, given the limitations of the particular circumstances. It is the responsibility of the consultant to provide feedback and guidance on the basis of the information provided, which is within his/her broad range of expertise, and which might be provided by, or recognized as reasonable, by a professional peer. This does not mean that the practitioner's peers would necessarily offer the same feedback, simply that the feedback is recognized as theoretically sound and "psychologically plausible".

'A consultation on the OPD pathway should always hold in mind the needs of the offender manager who is consulting as the primary concern, and should be relevant to the OM's remit within the Criminal Justice System' (personal communication, J Craissati).

Co-working is the only element that involves direct contact between the psychological therapist or PDPO and the offender, although this contact was always carried out in collaboration and in the presence of the supervising offender manager. Essentially, co-working comprised offering between one and six sessions—most commonly one or two—in order to overcome an impasse. This impasse took many forms, including:

- A breakdown in the relationship between the offender and the offender manager that held the possibility of repair

- An attempt to re-engage an offender in contemplating his pathway to the community (including the consideration of treatment) which he had previously rejected

- Reviewing the risk assessment in the light of agency or practitioner conflicting views

- Developing a formulation of a complex offender to build the confidence of the offender manager in collaborating on this task with the offender.

Approved Premises

In England and Wales, the National Probation Service (NPS) has access to a limited range of 24/7 supported hostel accommodation for offenders, referred to as Approved Premises (APs). Demand is inevitably higher than supply, and therefore places are reserved for those who pose a high risk of harm; placements are notionally for three months, although in reality many offenders with the most complex needs stay several months longer. Many of the OPD pathway offenders will have been released into the community having served lengthy custodial sentences. The APs therefore serve a dual function of enabling management of the risk posed by offenders, while providing a structured and supportive environment.

It was felt to be beneficial to provide an enhanced service to the pathway offenders placed in the twelve APs in London, and an opportunity to target services with potential for enhancing the impact of our intervention. This was particularly pertinent given the high rate of recalls—and other types of failure on post-custodial licence, including offending, associated with personality dysfunction. For example, a particularly high number of recalls (24%) occur in the first thirty days post-release [22]; an evaluation of a specialist AP for personality disordered offenders found that just over a third failed whilst resident. Psychopathy, self-defeating traits, and negative comments written in their records were predictors of failure [23].

The LPP worked with the NPS in London to deliver the following service: each AP team was released for six days' training, delivered over the course of two months. This included three days of personality disorder awareness training and three days of skills development (drawn from a range of perspectives, including dialectical behaviour therapy and attachment). The community specialist team then offered a weekly or fortnightly visit to each AP, and worked with the team on case consultation, formulation, and ongoing plans to manage challenging behaviours.

The LPP conducted an internal evaluation of the AP service, comparing the six hostels receiving the intervention first with the six hostels on a 'waiting list', and examining outcomes twelve months later. Most staff completed the questionnaires at at least one time point, but there was considerable drop-off over time, with staff movement in and out of the service. Two key staff questionnaires were used to measure confidence and competence in working with personality disorder (Personality Disorder—Knowledge Attitudes and Skills Questionnaire (PD-KASQ)) and burnout (Maslack Burnout Inventory). The Essen Climate Evaluation Schema (EssenCES) and Team Climate Inventory (short version) were also used.

The evaluation was able to demonstrate a significant improvement in staff self-reported confidence and competence regarding personality disorder, a reduction in emotional exhaustion, and improvement in personal accomplishment; and staff perceptions of the social therapeutic atmosphere of the AP were significantly superior in the experimental condition. The changes were sustained over an eighteen-month period. In terms of offender outcomes, planned move on to independent accommodation was evaluated, as well as failures including re-arrests and recalls to prison. Overall, 35% of the residents moved on in a mutually agreed fashion; however, of the remainder, only 1% of the sample was re-arrested for a new offence. It is important to note that the evaluation was not able to establish any discernible impact on these 'hard' outcomes; anecdotally, staff reported the recall rate as subject to issues outside their control, such as the presence of drugs in the APs or gang-related concerns [24].

Treatment

We decided on three options for the LPP delivery as part of the OPD community pathway, one of which was a stand-alone treatment approach and two were examples of integrated models of partnership working:

Stand-alone treatment approach

A pre-existing stand-alone treatment approach was available in South London, delivered separately by two of the four consortium trusts. One had been offering a slightly higher-cost, low-volume intensive approach to case management and treatment since 2005; the other service offered a lower-cost, higher-volume extended assessment and a psycho-educational group-work service which had grown over a period of two decades.

It became clear, as the core tasks were implemented across the whole of London, to what extent experienced community forensic psychological therapy services were able to support and enhance the delivery of the core tasks. At any one point in time, an estimated 100 OPD pathway offenders might have been held on the health caseloads of the two trusts, and the psychologists were able to respond to the anxieties of our third-sector partners (see section "Third-sector ('value-added') partnerships") and take on offenders who were coming to the end of their period of supervision. The combined mix of approaches—case management, brief engagement, psycho-educational workshops, and longer-term therapy—enabled engagement with a wide range of personality disordered offenders.

Mentalization-Based Therapy programme

The aim of MBT is to improve patients' capacity to 'mentalize'. Mentalizing is the process of holding your own mind in mind, while also attending to what may be going on in the mind of others. The development of MBT as a treatment for ASPD followed the pioneering work conducted by Bateman et al. [25] which was originally conceived and implemented as a treatment for BPD. Building on their initial work, more recent research has shown that MBT becomes even more effective with patients with multiple comorbid personality disorder diagnoses, and that only relatively minor adaptations are required to provide an intervention aimed at individuals with ASPD.

Failing to mentalize leads to marked difficulties in maintaining self-identity and affect regulation and impulsivity. A positive outcome of treatment would therefore be an increased ability to mentalize, which, it is hypothesized, will enhance the patient's ability to manage complex interpersonal and social situations and relationships. MBT has a range of techniques which the therapist uses to work with the patient's style of thinking and feeling. These techniques seek to encourage patients to reflect on the assumptions they make about others that may result in problematic and harmful behaviour, either to themselves or to others.

MBT is currently being provided across four London sites (fourteen sites in total across England and Wales) that form part of a national project to conduct a randomized controlled trial of the effectiveness of the programme across all the sites.

In order to meet the standards required to undertake the random controlled trial it has been necessary to impose a number of selection requirements for entry to the programme. Eligibility is restricted to men aged twenty one or over with a recent history of violence and a diagnosis of ASPD. They must be currently under the supervision of the NPS and have at least six months left on their licence. Offenders with a diagnosis of active psychosis, those who are dependent on alcohol and drugs, and those who have a history of child sex offending are excluded from the programme. The MBT programme is de-livered within probation premises by a dedicated part-time team comprised of three MBT therapists, with input from a PDPO and a service user. The group is a rolling programme, with participants joining as vacancies arise. Group members are expected to remain in the group for one year and are required to commit to both the weekly seventy-five-minute group therapy sessions and monthly individual sessions. Each group session is facilitated by two members of the staff team, and sessions are recorded and reviewed in order to monitor treatment efficacy.

In addition to the professional staff team, an innovative feature of MBT is the involvement of those with 'lived experience'. These individuals are ex-service users who themselves have a diagnosis of personality disorder and have suc-cessfully emerged through forensic systems. Each group employs, on a paid basis, at least one ex-service user who actively assists by co-facilitating the group. Initially, anxieties were raised regarding the participation of ex-service users for a number of reasons, including, for example, confidentiality. However, these concerns have not been borne out by experience, and feedback from par-ticipants has been overwhelmingly positive as they tend to view the ex-service users as having a greater level of understanding of the pressures and difficulties they routinely encounter compared to professional staff.

The randomized controlled trial has inevitably reduced the potential pool of possible participants, and recruitment to the programme has been very slow. This problem has been exacerbated by the high recall rate to prison of of-fenders with antisocial traits, on account of their rule-breaking and impulsive behaviours. Other, more complex issues arise due to the inherent difficulties in attempting to provide psychological intervention to this client group. There are many reasons why high-risk, antisocial individuals who have histories of acting out serious violence have traditionally been excluded from most community-based therapeutic provision. Many of their interpersonal difficulties arise because of their low tolerance to environmental stress and their tendency to apply a very limited range of rigid 'rules' in managing their relationships with others. Displays of aggressive anger or resorting to substance abuse are often means to resolve or avoid becoming overwhelmed by interpersonal anxiety. Often their violence or other forms of acting-out are triggered as a psychological defence against feelings of shame or humiliation at points when their view of themselves or the world is perceived to be undermined. Some form of acting-out as a method of avoiding emotional distress is therefore a common if not ubiquitous feature of ASPD, and one particularly prevalent form is dropping out of the group in response to feeling challenged in some way. Ensuring that robust governance procedures are in place to ensure the safety of the team and group members is essential if difficult issues are to be discussed within the group.

Challenge Project programme for high-risk sex offenders

The Challenge Project has been in operation in South East London for more than twenty years, initially as a partially integrated partnership with probation. With ongoing evaluation, it became clear that the programme was only effective with the higher-risk sex offenders, and it became increasingly focused on high-risk personality disordered offenders [9]. The programme is now delivered as part of the OPD pathway, and has been extended to cover the whole of London, with two groups running—one in North and one in South London.

The Challenge Project operates a similar structure to MBT, with weekly group work of two hours and less-intensive individual work, offered flexibly according to need. Criteria for entry include a contact sex offence (with either an adult or child victim) and at least two of the following: high risk of future sexual reoffending as measured by standardized tools, a substantive history of mental health contact, previous refusal to participate in treatment, failure in the form of reconviction following completion of previous treatment, or a history of significant behavioural problems. The therapeutic model pays attention to the important role that early attachments, trauma experiences, and failure to 'mentalize' play in the trajectory of offending; these ideas are integrated with more traditional cognitive behavioural approaches which explore the sexual assault cycle, decision making, and a 'good lives' approach to relapse prevention. The three-day maintenance programme runs for three consecutive days twice a year, and the highest-risk offenders are invited to opt in on an annual or biannual basis. The overall programme is manualized and therefore run in an identical manner in both sites.

The project has been repeatedly evaluated: most recently [8], participants were followed up for almost four years: 35% of the treatment participants had severe personality difficulties in two or more clusters; over 50% were high risk on static and dynamic risk tools; and 25% scored > 13 on the Psychopathy Checklist (short version). In terms of outcomes, 75% completed treatment without incident, even when attending voluntarily; 11% sexually reoffended (this dropped to 9% if non-completers were excluded); and 3% reoffended violently. This compares very favourably with expected rates.

Third-sector 'value-added' partnerships

We chose to include funding for third-sector partnerships in our bid, which might add value to the OPD pathway in London; these were based on the parallel partnership model. Our criteria for selection included:

- A track record in delivering innovative services to socially excluded individuals
- An explicitly stated appetite and capacity for working with complexity and risk
- Clearly fulfilling a need in terms of personality disordered offenders in areas where they might otherwise be excluded.

We commissioned three projects, which are detailed below.

SOVA Support Link

SOVA Support Link (SSL) was initially a project for one of the participating trusts in South East London, but expanded to cover all of London. It draws on the principles of COSA, which were first developed in Canada in the mid-1990s based on the principles of restorative justice (described in the section 'Management approaches' [14]).

SSL aims to assist offenders on the personality disorder pathway build supportive social networks in which they experience themselves as active agents, and to consolidate and develop their own resources and improve quality of life. The model views enhancement of offenders' well-being and reduction of their risk of further offending as inextricably linked, and suggests that the best way to create a safer society is, therefore, to assist offenders to adopt a more fulfilling and socially integrated lifestyle. SSL volunteers are recruited from local communities and are thus in a position to contribute to breaking down myths and stereotypes around offending, especially sexual offending, which in turn contribute to stigmatization and social exclusion of individuals with offending histories. To sustain desistance from crime, the person who has criminal convictions must find a new identity and meaningful role within civil society—and this requires reciprocity and recognition from the community. The idea is to promote psychological well-being through building positive relationships which sustain and nurture hope, increase opportunities for social inclusion, reduce social loneliness, and improve quality of life.

The project is subject to ongoing evaluation. However, the first twenty participants of the service were evaluated on a range of quantitative and qualitative measures before and after the intervention, and followed up for a further year [26]. The sample size was small, but in general the findings were cautiously encouraging. That is, self-reported quality of life and social/emotional loneliness improved; engagement levels were high; and of 77 goals identified, around 70% were either fully or partially achieved. Rates of self-harm and substance misuse improved, and participants were maintained in their independent accommodation.

First Step Trust work project

First Step Trust (FST) provides training and work experience opportunities for up to twenty personality disorder pathway offenders who otherwise would be excluded from mainstream employment services. Workforce members take on the responsibilities and pressures of real work, in an environment that is supportive and understanding of their needs. The aim of the service is to help workforce members address the issues and challenges facing them by becoming less dependent on health and social care services, and to assist with their transition away from offending behaviour. Opportunities include garage mechanics, office working, garden maintenance, and painting and decorating.

The reality is that few of the offenders are work ready, and many are overwhelmed by chaos in their everyday lives, suspicious of others' motives, and entangled in complex difficulties with the social security system which pays their benefits. FST offers supervision throughout the day, which is the key element allowing risk to the public to be managed, and a careful balance between the development of appropriate work-related boundaries (for example, no talking about offences at any point during the day) and a flexible and compassionate response to ambivalent engagement.

Women in Prison

Women in Prison is in partnership with the LPP in order to provide a case management service for fifteen women offenders who are identified as part of the OPD pathway in London and are being released into the community from custody. Each woman accepted into the service receives support from a complex-needs, through-the-gate worker who provides emotional and practical resettlement support on a range of issues (mental health, housing, domestic violence, substance use, benefits, education and training, family and parenting) to women in custody. Following their release to the community, clients are assisted in their engagement with both statutory (community mental health teams, general practitioners (GPs), social services, probation) and non-statutory (voluntary sector) services, and to manage their appointments.

Observations of the third-sector partnerships

There is no doubt that our third-sector partnerships brought innovation and energy to the LPP, as well as being well regarded by the service users. However—as with other aspects of the pathway—it has been a challenge to quantify the impact of their contribution on the higher-level outcomes. Our experience is that participating service users largely forge mutually gratifying relationships with the services which endure; but they do not succeed in transferring these relationships to the wider community. Jobs are not available, relationships are not forthcoming, they have been left behind by their pro-social peer group, and shared interests cannot be pursued because of the fear of third-party disclosure.

All three projects also struggled with their expansion from a small, local, and intimate service to a London-wide delivery. The very elements that made them so successful in their locality were very bound up with a leadership style that was sympathetic to our model, and predicated on a close and mutually supportive relationship between the partners. With growth, the influence of the project leads diminished, in some cases skills were diluted with the expansion of the staff team, and in all cases impact suffered as a result of geographically dispersed service users. Over time, it became clear just how important the project lead was in promoting and maintaining the understanding of the partnership model, and the core aim of each project; without strong and very visible leadership, the projects were pulled—to a greater or lesser extent—towards their generic service model—returning to doing what they usually do. Broadly speaking, the projects were excellent at engaging the more vulnerable and isolated offenders or those who tended to seek out services, albeit in a rather chaotic fashion; the projects were less successful with highly antisocial individuals who were reluctant to own their difficulties or accept assistance.

Evaluation

Evaluation of specific elements of the community pathway has been described earlier in this chapter (see, for example, the section on 'Approved Premises', 'The

Challenge Project programme for high-risk sex offenders', or 'SOVA Support Link'). A London-wide, externally commissioned evaluation has now been completed [27, 28] and contains a detailed analysis of all elements of the core tasks. In summary, the evaluation confirmed the approximate figures detailed in Fig. 4.1, and provided additional detail:

♦ Appropriately high-risk offenders were being targeted for consideration, and these offenders were making progress along the pathway, for both men and women.

♦ The OPD screening was capturing a higher proportion of black and minority ethnic groups than other screening methods, but these individuals were not progressing as robustly as white British offenders along the pathway.

♦ Recommendations for progression were only followed up by actual referrals in around 35% of cases.

♦ When compared to a matched comparison group, high-risk offenders in the pathway showed a significantly greater desirable change in their dynamic risk rating for general offending, but not for violent offending; this was also true of medium-risk offenders, when matched to a control group. Furthermore, offenders in the pathway who were low risk for further violence on the basis of a criminogenic score were more likely to remain low risk than their matched controls. However, the overall picture was that the OPD pathway in London was not necessarily resulting in a consistent lowering of the risk profile or risk concerns, as measured by the probation tool the Offender Assessment System (OASys).

Reflections three years on, and next steps

Matters out of our control

The community pathway has been able to maintain control over certain factors (e.g. the specific model of operation). There have, however, been a range of sometimes unforeseen external factors in response to which there has been no alternative but to accept, embrace, and adapt working practice in a flexible manner. One of the most important of these external changes was the TR programme that took place in June 2014 when the community pathway was still in its infancy [29]. TR was a hugely significant change to the way that probation services were provided across England and Wales, resulting in a separation of the probation service into that delivered for high-risk cases (approximately 30% of the total caseload), which from that point onwards was exclusively managed within the NPS, while all low- and medium-risk cases (approximately 70% of the total) were transferred to the newly created CRC, which was run by a newly appointed American company, MTCnovo.

Probation staff were allocated to work in either NPS or CRC. This resulted in a huge reallocation of cases, and during that initial phase there were many offender managers who had little knowledge of the offenders on their caseload. Many long-standing working relationships that had been built up, sometimes over many years, between offenders and particular officers were broken (as were working relationships between staff). This change was resisted by many individuals working in the probation service and had a major detrimental impact on probation staff morale (see Box 4.2).

The ripples of this low morale were felt across the community pathway, with a general sense of offender managers having little interest in investing time and energy into trying something new at a time of such fundamental systemic change. OPD pathway staff struggled to engage their colleagues, at a time when achieving progress in training and consultation key performance indicators (KPIs) had become paramount.

There were, however, a number of benefits arising from these changes in streamlining our work in the community pathway. Because the high-risk cases were concentrated onto the caseloads of fewer staff, this reduced the number of staff with whom it was necessary to consult and provide training. Each offender manager subsequently had a greater proportion of screened-in cases with which they were working, increasing their exposure, skills, and confidence when working with the difficulties associated with the client group.

At the frontline of this interface between health and probation is the working relationship between the psychological therapist and the specialist offender manager within each LDU. Together, these two professionals are accountable for the delivery of the pathway at the local level. It is inevitable that the respective professional ethos and background of the two different organizations

Box 4.2 Transforming rehabilitation—a case example

'I don't have time to attend the reflective practice group; I've got to get to grips with a whole new caseload—it keeps changing, and they're all high risk. Team members keep going off to other jobs or they're sick or something, the pressure is enormous. And there's so much tension in the office—you wouldn't believe it but I can't sit on chairs that belong to the CRC (sharing an office)! Management don't seem to know much more than us.' Offender manager.

(health and probation) and any tensions that might exist between these organizations will be replicated in the relationship between staff on the frontline. The organizational priorities to which each organization is subject will inevitably emerge in the working relationship between these two individuals.

Feeling more out of control

For the psychological therapists employed as part of the community pathway, working within probation settings provides a different set of challenges than they are likely to encounter in what might be considered more 'traditional' environments, such as health or prison settings. In such settings, it is common for psychologists to be one member of a larger multi-disciplinary team in which each professional contributes to the decision-making process. Many of the psychological therapists engaged in community pathways work will be relatively early in their careers and may not have had extensive experience of working directly with personality disordered offenders. Although they may hold specialist academic knowledge in regard to personality disorder and be very skilled at developing psychological formulations, having the ability to effectively communicate that knowledge to a staff group from a different professional background, and whose willingness to positively embrace change may have been undermined by external changes beyond their control, has at times proven to require a high level of persistence and creativity. Overall, community pathway work requires the psychologist to have not just a sufficient level of knowledge, but also the required confidence to work autonomously in order to provide consultation to colleagues from a different professional background, whose training and practice is based upon quite different core principles and assumptions (see Box 4.3).

PDPOs will also find that pathways work has many differences from the tasks to which they will have become accustomed as part of their everyday supervision of offenders. They are unlikely to have had previous experience in providing consultation, and, in addition, since the PDPOs are drawn from the local office in which they are already based, they are faced with the added task of renegotiating relationships with colleagues with whom they may have previously worked for a considerable period but in a very different capacity. There may be concerns about precisely what it means to be viewed as a specialist who holds additional knowledge. Furthermore, we have noted that developing reflective skills and learning to understand complex cases from a more psychologically oriented perspective brings difficulties as well as benefits; defences which provide resilience—for example, a somewhat detached approach, a focus on risk rather than the person, the simple imposition of standardized rules—are broken down, with greater levels of ambiguity and ambivalence taking their

Box 4.3 The challenges of partnership working—a case example

An offender manager made a complaint regarding the local psychological therapist for the OPD pathway, expressing resentment that she was overly interfering in his management of a tricky case; he maintained she was dogmatic and unrealistic in her expectations. The psychological therapist, qualified within the past year, was defensive in her response, pointing out that the offender manager was insufficiently responsive to this particular offender's clinical needs. This interpersonal dynamic reflected the difficulties of the pathway—an anxious clinician overcompensating for feelings of inadequacy and focusing more on her area of competence than the needs of the offender manager (who in turn felt rather exposed and threatened by her involvement).

place. This may inadvertently render the work more not less complex, and expose the practitioner's vulnerabilities.

The partnership, at local-delivery level, also struggled at times with the tendency to pull back into traditional expert consultant-dependent consultee roles. This sometimes resulted in probation officers relying on the psychological therapist's formulation, without fully assimilating it into their own thinking. Reversion to more traditional health versus criminal justice preoccupations (care versus control) was also a tension that had to be overcome by working at the relationships within the partnership.

Trying to regain control

Perhaps the greatest area of learning was the difficulty of generalizing from a small successful pilot in one area to a pan-London delivery. This is an unexceptional observation, but nevertheless a real one, particularly at a time of political upheaval. This challenge is best exemplified by our struggle to achieve a consistent service across every area, as measured by the presence of a collaborative probation and health team, near 100% case identification, regular case consultation, and formulations for those appearing to have the most pressing need. Data monitoring exposed differences in performance; practitioners had very different experiences of a competitively tendered service, and what might be expected from the commissioners; the leaders varied in their approach to managing performance. Eventually we introduced a formal rating system: a 'traffic-light' system was developed to monitor performance of each borough against KPIs. Areas working well and meeting most if not all targets are rated green. Areas in which there are less serious problems but which still require attention are rated amber. More serious problems, which might include long-term unfilled vacancies or persistent failure to progress on the KPIs are rated red, allowing those boroughs to be prioritized by developing a detailed plan to address the difficulties.

Implementing this performance model in response to difficulties led to a period of acrimony, coming as it did at a time of low morale. Acrimony took the form of quibbles regarding the accuracy of data and ratings, with challenges and counter challenges as to who was most at fault. With a little more attention paid to repairing the relationship, the situation settled. Clearly, with hindsight, it would have been preferable to anticipate difficulties in advance and agree a monitoring system before tensions set in. Nevertheless, the model is now embedded in the delivery of the service, accompanied by very timely and regular local updates of performance and progress on key targets, which enables local-delivery practitioners to shift their focus as required.

Summary and next steps

To summarize where we are now, over the course of three years, London now has:

- A consortium of four mental health trusts working cordially in partnership to share delivery of the OPD pathway
- Psychological therapists located in partnership with PDPOs in every local area across London, offering an identical service no matter where an offender resides
- Psychological support to all twelve approved premises (hostels for probation)
- All cases are screened for personality disorder, and where there are complex issues, discussions have taken place and formulations written down
- More recently, two Intensive Intervention and Risk Management Services (IIRMS) have been established in London, allowing offenders who are screened in and resident in the community greater access to interventions.

This progress is mirrored nationally—no small achievement over the past three years. In 2017, the community OPD pathway specification was reviewed and additional guidance provided to practitioners. There are no further revisions planned for the foreseeable future.

Locally, we now have to focus on ensuring that the service—spread thinly as it is—maximizes its impact in terms of the OPD pathway high-level outcomes. Levels of recall to prison remain a concern—albeit not entirely in our control—and we need to monitor and learn from all failures. It is also important to ensure that we can argue the economic as well as the social benefits of progressing high-risk offenders through the system. A preliminary audit of progress in those cases where the team has provided formulations and advice suggests that in the first two years we were responsible for 600 offenders being accepted by a range of intervention services, with 350 having started in the new service and 100 having completed. The results from the pilot phase of the community programme also demonstrated a significant impact on outcomes, in terms of those offenders who had had contact with the OPD pathway psychologists having a lower failure rate (in terms of recall or reoffending) in the community than those who had had no contact [30]. This is an encouraging start to an ambitious project.

There are probably two priority areas for the London OPD pathway service in the next two years; we think it likely that these priorities will resonate with other OPD services across England and Wales. First is the need for the service to enhance its observable impact on outcomes, and to evidence this. That is, the sheer size of the task absorbed the teams' energy in the first few years, and there are now opportunities to shift the focus of work to ensuring that prisoners keep progressing and that community failures are reduced to a healthy minimum. Second, access to evidence-based personality disorder interventions and enhanced case management has expanded over the past year, but there continues to be an uneven delivery of interventions across the Greater London area; our aim is to ensure that all offenders in the city have equal access to an appropriate range of services.

References

1. **Bedics JD, Atkins DC, Harned MS, Linehan MM.** The therapeutic alliance as a predictor of outcome in dialectical behaviour therapy versus nonbehavioural psychotherapy by experts for borderline personality disorder. Psychotherapy. 2015;**52**(1):67–77.

2. **Davidson KM.** Cognitive therapy for personality disorders: a guide for clinicians, 2nd edn. Hove: Routledge; 2008.

3. **Hollin CR, McGuire J, Hounsome J, Hatcher R, Bilby C, Palmer EJ.** Cognitive skills offending behaviour programmes in the community: A reconviction analysis. Criminal Justice and Behaviour. 2008;**35**:269–283.

4. **McMurran M, Theodosi E.** Is treatment non-completion associated with increased reconviction over no treatment? Psychology, Crime and Law. 2007;**13**(4):333–343.

5. **Marques JK, Wiederanders M, Day DM, Nelson C, Van Ommeren A.** Effects of a relapse prevention program on sexual recidivism: final results from California's sex offender treatment and evaluation project (SOTEP). Sexual Abuse: A Journal of Research and Treatment. 2005;**17**:79–107.

6. **McGuire J.** A review of effective interventions for reducing aggression and violence. Philosophical Transactions of the Royal Society London. Series B. Biological Sciences. 2008;**363**:2577–2597.

7. **McGuire J.** 'What works' to reduce re-offending: 18 years on. In LA Craig, L Dixon, and TA Gannon (Eds.), What works in offender rehabilitation: an evidence-based approach to assessment and treatment. Chichester: Wiley-Blackwell; 2013, pp. 20–49.

8. **Craissati J, Blundell R.** A community service for high-risk mentally disordered sex offenders: A follow-up study. Journal of Interpersonal Violence. 2013;**28**(6):1178–1200.

9. **Tyrer P, Mulder R.** Management of complex and severe personality disorders in community mental health services. Current Opinion in Psychiatry. 2006;**19**:400–404.

10. **Home Office.** Joint inspection report into persistent and prolific offenders. London: Home Office Communications Directorate; 2004.

11. Livesley WJ, Dimaggio G, Clarkin JF (Eds.). Integrated treatment for personality disorder. New York: The Guilford Press; 2016.

12. **Peck M.** Patterns of reconviction among offenders eligible for MAPPA. London: Ministry of Justice; 2011.

13. **Hood R, Shute S.** Parole decision-making: weighing the risk to the public. Home Office Research Findings No. 114. London: Home Office; 2000.

14. **Bates A, Macrae R, Williams D, Webb C.** Ever-increasing circles: a descriptive study of Hampshire and Thames Valley circles of support and accountability 2002–2009. Journal of Sexual Aggression. 2011;**18**:355–373.

15. **Wilson R, Picheca J, Prinzo M, Cortoni F.** Circles of support and accountability: engaging community volunteers in the management of high-risk sexual offenders. The Howard Journal. 2007;**46**:1–15.

16. **Hanvey S.** But does it work? Evaluation and evidence. In S Hanvey, T Philpot, and C Wilson (Eds.), A community based approach to the reduction of sexual reoffending. London: Jessica Kingsley; 2011.

17. **Ward M, Attwell P.** Evaluation of two community outreach forensic psychological services. Journal of Forensic Practice. 2014;**16**(4):312–326.

18. **Kemshall H, Wood J.** Child Sex Offender Review (CSOR). Public disclosure pilots: a process evaluation, second edition. Research Report 32: Key Findings. London: Home Office; 2010.

19. **Home Office.** Domestic violence disclosure scheme pilot assessment. London: Home Office; 2013. http://www.gov.uk/government/publications/ domestic-violence-disclosure-scheme-pilot-assessment.

20. **Dowsett J, Craissati J.** Managing personality disordered offenders in the community: a psychological approach. Abingdon: Taylor Francis; 2008.

21. **Davies R.** The inter-disciplinary network and the internal world of the offender. In C Cordess and M Cox (Eds.), Forensic psychotherapy: crime, psychodynamics and the offender patient. London: Jessica Kingsley; 1998, p. 133.

22. **National Association of Probation Officers.** Huge rise in recalls of dangerous prisoners. Briefing for the cross party justice unions' parliamentary group. London: National Association of Probation Officers; 2011.

23. **Blumenthal S, Craissati J, Minchin L.** The development of a specialist hostel for the community management of personality disordered offenders. Criminal Behaviour and Mental Health. 2009;**19**(1):43–53.

24. **Bruce M, Stevens P.** Evaluation of the LPP Approved Premise Intervention. Internal Report to Commissioners. London: LPP; 2016.

25. **Bateman A, Bolton R, Fonagy P.** Antisocial personality disorder: a mentalizing framework. Focus: Journal of Lifelong Learning in Psychiatry. 2013;**11**:1–9.

26. **Smith L, Attwell P, Connor S.** 'Better than therapy'. Supporting ex-offenders: an evaluation of a voluntary community project. Internal report. London: Sova; 2014.

27. **Jolliffe D, Cattell J, Raza A, Minoudis P.** Factors associated with progression in the London Pathway Project. Criminal Behaviour and Mental Health. 2017;**27**:222–237.

28. **Jolliffe D, Cattell J, Raza, A, Minoudis P.** Evaluating the impact of the London Pathway Project. Criminal Behaviour and Mental Health. 2017;**27**:238–253.

29. **Ministry of Justice.** Transforming Rehabilitation: a strategy for reform. London: Home Office; 2013.

30. **Minoudis P, Shaw J, Craissati J.** The London Pathways Project: evaluating the effectiveness of a consultation model for personality disordered offenders. Criminal Behaviour and Mental Health. 2012;**22**(3):218–232.

Chapter 5

Intervening in secure settings

Colin Campbell and Pamela Attwell

Introduction

There have been services in UK prisons for offenders with personality disorder for decades. In addition to widely available offending behaviour programmes, there have been a small number of treatment services, most notably the therapeutic community (TC) in HMP Grendon and the Special Unit in Barlinnie Prison. However, these services tended to be isolated centres of good practice, often aimed at specific subpopulations of personality disordered offenders, based on offence type and motivation to engage in treatment. They were unable to integrate into a broader network of similar services and their lack of scale made it difficult to effectively evaluate the interventions used. With the advent of the Dangerous and Severe Personality Disorder (DSPD) programme, new prison services were developed with a clear focus on providing treatment for the highest-risk offenders; skilling up a workforce to deliver these services; and evaluating the interventions to establish what worked. However, it is the implementation of the Offender Personality Disorder (OPD) strategy in 2011 that represents the most significant change in prison services for personality disordered offenders. Building on the experience of the prison DSPD services, there has been a clear shift from health-based services to provision within prisons, with a national network of services tailored to meet the diverse treatment, risk, and responsivity needs of this population, from the point of conviction through to release and supervision in the community.

This chapter begins by reviewing the evidence base for services for offenders with personality disorder in secure settings and outlines the approaches used outside of the UK. It then sets out the commissioning context of the OPD pathway secure services, including the constraints, and why the London Pathways Partnership (LPP) took the approach it did. This is followed by a more detailed outline of how the services were delivered, from development through to evaluation, with consideration of what worked and what could have worked better. The chapter concludes with some suggestions for future directions in secure services for this group of offenders.

Secure services for personality disordered offenders

Prison services

Mainstream prison services have traditionally offered psychologically informed interventions at broadly three levels of intensity: accredited offending behaviour programmes, TCs, and high-secure specialist personality disorder units.

Offending behaviour programmes

Since the late 1990s, there has been a shift from a 'nothing works' position in relation to both interventions for offenders and treatment for individuals with personality disorder. Meta-analytic studies have demonstrated that interventions with offenders do reduce offending behaviour (e.g. [1, 2]), and personality disorder is no longer seen as 'untreatable'.

A wide range of Her Majesty's Prison and Probation Service (HMPPS) accredited offending behaviour programmes are available within the prison establishment. These programmes have an international reputation for large-scale delivery of offence-relevant, manualized interventions, delivered by semi-qualified staff.

These interventions tend to address specific offence or problem types, for example, violence, substance misuse, and sexual offending, and are of short to medium duration. The most effective tend to be cognitive behavioural interventions that allow for allocation of individuals to different levels of intervention according to their likely risk. However, most programmes are intended for medium- and high-risk individuals. Offending behaviour programmes are underpinned by the Risk, Needs, Responsivity (RNR) model, which was developed by Andrews, Bonta, and Hodge [3]. Offenders with the highest risk level are delivered the highest level of intervention, and dynamic risk factors ('criminogenic needs') are prioritized as a focus for intervention.

Effective interventions are likely to be highly structured, delivered by enthusiastic and appropriately trained staff, and carried out with high-risk offenders. The first national evaluation of the impact of cognitive skills programmes was encouraging [4], and there is evidence of good outcome for programmes based on the principles of RNR [5]. However, evidence for cognitive behavioural offending behaviour programmes in the UK remains mixed and study designs have made it difficult to attribute any positive impact on reoffending to the treatment or intervention itself, rather than other factors such as motivation to engage [6].

These mainstream offending behaviour programmes may, however, not be suitable for all offenders, and offenders with severe personality disorder have been shown to be less able to benefit from them [7, 8]. They may not have accessed the programmes due to personality difficulties or related exclusion criteria. It is also likely that aspects of dysfunctional personality interfere with completing accredited programmes, so that personality disorder is over-represented in those who fail to complete programmes [9]. Individuals with severe personality disorder are also more likely to struggle with consolidation of what is learned and with periods of transition and/or progress. More intensive work on their complex interpersonal needs may need to be completed first, or conjointly with these programmes. In addition to difficulties completing treatment and sustaining treatment gains, offenders with personality disorder may be deficient in qualities that have been highlighted by the desistance literature as contributing to reintegration into the community and long-term desistance from crime: for example, a sense of personal agency, self-control, belief in personal self-efficacy, and a new self-narrative.

Democratic therapeutic communities

The Henderson Hospital, founded in 1947, was the first established TC in England. TCs are essentially a social treatment milieu, characterized by an informal atmosphere, regular meetings, and participation in running the community. The first TC located in a prison setting opened in HMP Grendon in 1962, and Grendon remains the only prison in England that serves as a pure TC.

Democratic TCs (DTCs) provide a long-term, intensive, residential offending behaviour intervention for prisoners with complex needs, many of whom have moderate to severe personality disorder. The degree of need in these prisoners may prevent them from benefitting from shorter interventions, and prisoners are expected to stay for at least eighteen months to give them sufficient time to learn from the experience and consolidate new skills through practice. There are at the time of writing fourteen DTCs (three of which are newly developed TC+s, modified for learning disabled offenders) across five prisons.

In prisons, the DTCs provide a 'living-learning' environment with a specific focus on the supportive and challenging network of relationships between members of the community. TC residents participate in group therapy, where they openly explore their offending behaviour and encourage other group members to do the same. Weekly community meetings chaired by a prisoner and underpinned by a constitution provide a forum for the community to regulate itself. TC residents will also work, attend education, and may attend other complementary programmes and therapies. The assumption is that optimal functioning within the TC promotes better functioning in other settings [10]. However, the TC milieu is very specific and differs from the realities of the outside world or general setting in prison.

There is a growing evidence base for the impact of TCs on both psychological well-being and reoffending. A meta-analysis of twenty nine studies of both democratic and hierarchical TC effectiveness found a strong positive effect for TC treatment [11]. Evaluation of the TC at HMP Grendon has shown that prisoners have a more positive view of their quality of life than other prisoners and that staff perceive the social climate to be more positive than in other secure settings. Following treatment, residents experience lower levels of anxiety and depression and are less hostile and negative, with fewer negative relating tendencies. Importantly, residents serving life sentences who stay in therapy for eighteen months are also less likely to be reconvicted than prisoners selected for Grendon but who do not come to the service [12].

DTCs may not, however, be suitable for all personality disordered offenders. Residents need to be reasonably psychologically minded and to be motivated to engage in what can be challenging treatment. Those who find it difficult to manage transition and to engage with an unfamiliar team may struggle to engage with the referral and assessment process, which could result in them being deemed unsuitable. Drop-out rates are not insignificant and, of those who do complete eighteen months of treatment, many struggle with progression from the unit and to 'recover' from leaving the service.

Former DSPD services

Prior to the development of the OPD strategy, treatment services were delivered for personality disordered offenders in two high-secure prisons as part of the DSPD programme (see Chapter 1). These services, one in the north and one in the south of England, have now been incorporated into the OPD pathway.

Treatment in the first service is based on a cognitive interpersonal model and is delivered through both individual therapy and a progressive programme of group work, which initially focuses on affective and interpersonal dysfunction before moving on to offending behaviour, addictive behaviours, and healthy relationships.

The Chromis programme is an accredited programme delivered in the second of the two units. This programme has been specially designed to address risk of violence in men whose high levels of psychopathic traits disrupt their ability to engage in treatment and maintain change. Participants begin by completing the first of five treatment components, which focuses on motivation and engagement, followed by further components on creative thinking, problem solving, handling conflict, and cognitive self-change. There is some evidence that the programme has a positive impact on some intermediate and process outcomes. For example, Tew and Atkinson [13] found that completion of Chromis has been linked to some reduction in self-reported anger and improved institutional behaviour, such as a reduction in expected incidents of physical aggression within custody. It is, however, possible that these findings reflect the impact of the Westgate Unit regime as a whole, as opposed to the Chromis programme specifically.

Due to their location in the high-secure estate, former prison DSPD services focus on category A and B prisoners. They also tend to have more specific entry criteria in terms of personality disorder diagnosis, in terms of specific traits, such as psychopathic traits, or complexity. Participants also need to have a reasonable degree of motivation to engage in treatment, which may last for at least three to five years, and therefore must also have the required period left of their sentence to complete treatment. Arguably, such services are therefore better suited to men who are at an early stage in their sentence, and may present particular difficulties in terms of motivation to engage than men who are post-tariff or who have not been released at a recent Parole Board hearing.

Secure health services

With the expansion of services for personality disordered offenders in prison settings, there were parallel developments in hospital-based services. The focus of these services in the UK has largely been the high-secure, or 'special', hospitals. Many of the patients admitted to the new Broadmoor Criminal Lunatic Asylum in the 1860s were diagnosed with 'moral insanity', more detailed clinical descriptions of which are consistent with a diagnosis of personality disorder. Services of one form or another have continued to be provided for patients with personality disorder in all three high-secure hospitals in England ever since. Although they have driven significant developments in the treatment and management of such patients, they have often been the focus of significant controversy. Several major public inquires have been highly critical of the management and delivery of these complex services and recommended the closure of one [14].

Innovation in non-forensic settings, both community and in-patient, also helped shape secure services for personality disordered offenders. These services were often built up around one or two clinicians who, with like-minded commissioners, were able to develop centres of excellence in the management of personality disorder. Evaluation of these services confirmed the effectiveness of some of the key elements underpinning current services for offenders, such as DTC principles and the combination of intensive in-patient treatment with outreach follow-up. In the 1990s, prior to the introduction of the DSPD programme, there were also a small number of services for offenders with personality disorder in medium-secure settings, most notably Arnold Lodge, but also in the independent sector.

Amongst the many drivers behind the DSPD programme, there was recognition that, although services existed in high-secure hospitals, the lack of services in medium security meant that there was no clear progression pathway for offenders with personality disorder. The proposal to develop services in a hospital setting also provided an option for prisoners approaching the end of determinate sentences, who had treatment needs related to personality disorder and who continued to pose a significant risk to others. It also meant that more specialist services would be available for individuals with personality disorder who were already detained under a hospital order, but who failed to progress in existing high-secure services.

As part of the DSPD programme, services were developed in two high-secure hospitals, together with three medium-secure and community services (see Chapter 1). Following evaluation of the DSPD programme and the introduction of the OPD strategy, one of the high-secure services was decommissioned and the decommissioning of the second service is proposed. With a focus on treatment and management in prison settings, it is envisaged that transfer to hospital should be for time-limited interventions for a specific subgroup of personality disordered offenders, with transfer back to one of the expanding number of prison services as the next progressive move in the pathway. This group of offenders includes those with complex comorbidity, intractable self-harm, and extremely challenging behaviour. However, although diminishing in number, secure health services also remain necessary for patients with personality disorder, who are given a hospital order, with or without restriction, at the time of sentencing.

International context

There is considerable variation internationally in the provision of services for personality disordered offenders within prisons. This is largely due to two factors. First, variations exist in criminal and mental health legislation between jurisdictions and how this facilitates diversion to hospital for treatment or to specialist services within the prison system. The second factor concerns attitudes regarding the treatability of personality disorder and the extent to which offenders with personality disorder are responsible for their offending behaviour, both of which are influenced by a range of social and political factors, as discussed in Chapter 1.

Legal definitions of mental disorder have historically been limited to psychotic disorders and there is considerable variation in the extent to which different jurisdictions include personality disorder [15]. For example, in the US, mental incapacity statutes explicitly exclude disorders characterized only by repeated criminal conduct. In some states, the definition is expanded to exclude individuals who solely have a personality disorder from eligibility for an insanity defence. In other jurisdictions, such as Canada, Belgium, and Germany, personality disorder is included but remains subject to considerable legal debate.

Following conviction, some countries, such as the Netherlands and Sweden, allow the option of indeterminate detention in a secure forensic hospital, subject to regular review of ongoing risk. Others, such as the US, Canada, and Australia, have community protection models, which allow civil commitment for indeterminate periods provided the offender continues to present a risk to the public. In the US, some states have Mentally Disordered Offender statutes, which provide a mechanism to detain mentally disordered offenders who reach the end of a determinate prison term and remain a risk to others as a result of a mental disorder. This legislation is largely used to civilly commit offenders with psychotic disorders. However, Sexually Violent Predator statutes allow for the civil commitment of sex offenders with a 'mental abnormality' following a prison sentence, where they are considered likely to engage in predatory acts of sexual violence if not detained in a secure environment [16]. 'Mental abnormality' is interpreted very broadly, and antisocial personality disorder and paraphilia not otherwise specified (NOS) are the most common diagnoses in this population.

Where transfer to services for personality disordered offenders is facilitated by the relevant legislation, resources are often limited and treatment models lack an evidence base for this population. Many services are developed for specific subpopulations of offenders, such as sexual offenders, which by default have a high prevalence of personality disorder. For example, most offenders in Social Therapeutic Institutions (STIs) in the German correctional system are sex offenders, and the treatment models are not specifically developed to treat personality disorder [17]. Although there is considerable variability in the treatment models used in STIs, most deliver group treatment with a focus on social skills training, empathy training, self-management, and health education.

Other services have been specifically developed to treat personality disorder that is associated with risk of offending behaviour. The Violence Reduction Programme in Canada and the Dutch Ter Beschikking Stelling (TBS) system in the Netherlands are described in Chapter 1. Another example is START NOW, a manualized, group-based coping skills therapy developed in the Connecticut Department of Corrections in the US. The programme is based on a cognitive behavioural framework and consists of thirty two sessions in four units: foundational; emotional management; interpersonal; and future focused. Evaluation of START NOW has shown an inverse dose-response relationship between the number of sessions completed and the number of disciplinary reports [18]. There is some evidence that offenders in the highest-security-risk groups benefit most from the programme and it has been shown to be effective for offenders with a range of psychiatric diagnoses.

Outside of these examples of best practice, services for offenders with personality disorder are either non-existent or characterized by lack of resources; inadequate identification of personality disorder; considerable variation in treatment models; lack of an evidence-base approach; and poor co-ordination and integration with community provision.

Commissioning of secure services

In contrast to OPD services in the community, where providers had a degree of flexibility in proposing how to deliver the key tasks of these services at a local level, secure services were defined by identified need at a national level. A series of specifications and service models were developed by the joint National Health Service England (NHSE)/HMPPS commissioners to meet these needs, with limited opportunity for providers to introduce much variation into these highly specified services.

Some of the options for providing services for personality disordered offenders in secure settings were excluded by the principles of the OPD strategy themselves (see Chapter 1). For example, the development of additional services in secure health settings would not be in keeping with the principles of shared responsibility, joint operations, or, clearly, being predominantly based in the criminal justice system. Other options were excluded because of existing provision elsewhere, such as DTCs, or because of current commissioning priorities and identified local need, for example services for women.

A key feature of all secure services was the focus on the role of the social environment in improving the quality of relationships. This emphasized the opportunities for offenders to implement new skills in a relational context and for positive reinforcement of meeting needs in a prosocial way. This focus was formalized in two approaches to secure services, namely Psychologically Informed Planned Environments (PIPEs) and Enabling Environments. The PIPE model was a non-negotiable framework for many secure services in a range of settings, and all secure services have to work towards achieving the Enabling Environment award.

Psychologically Informed Planned Environments

'PIPEs are defined as specifically designed, contained environments where staff members have additional training to develop an increased psychological understanding of their work' [19].

PIPEs can be prison wings or Approved Premises in the community. They provide a safe and supportive environment where there is a focus on the quality of staff/resident relationships and interactions. PIPEs are not a treatment, they are a living environment designed to support the offender's psychological well-being and encourage the practice and development of newly acquired prosocial skills and lifestyle choices. The aim is to reduce risk-related behaviours and enable offenders to progress through a pathway of intervention, consolidating skills that have previously been learned, and supporting transition and personal development at significant stages of their pathway.

The PIPE model originated as part of a response to the need for progression services for men and women who had completed intensive interventions, in particular the DSPD programme [20]. It is widely accepted that individuals with severe personality disorder may be destabilized by transitions or periods of change, and it was recognized that services designed to provide appropriate support at these times could contribute to stability and consolidation of gains made in therapeutic interventions.

All PIPE services focus on psychosocial relating and aim to improve social integration and social functioning. They all have a focus on the experience of transition, irrespective of in which part of the pathway they are located. They all share the six core components outlined below [20]. However, there are also significant differences between PIPEs, dependent on which population they serve and where along the pathway they are located. These differences are described after the core components of all PIPEs have been identified.

Core components

There are six core components to the PIPE model, described briefly below:

- *Enabling Environment*: each PIPE service is required to work towards the Enabling Environment award, which has been developed and validated by the Royal College of Psychiatrists (see section on 'Enabling Environments' for more details).

- *Workforce development*: the training and development of staff is a critical component of the PIPE model delivery. All staff are trained in working with people with personality disorder, undertaking the Knowledge and Understanding Framework awareness level as a minimum (see Chapter 2). Staff also receive training on the creation of an Enabling Environment and working with and understanding groups.

- *Staff supervision*: all staff are required to participate in both group and individual supervision processes. Individual clinical supervision for operational staff is usually facilitated by the Clinical Leads, and group supervision for operational and clinical staff may be facilitated by the Clinical Lead or, ideally, an external facilitator who has a good understanding of the PIPE model. The model of supervision follows a group analytic approach, described by Brown [21], in which each of the Clinical Leads is supported by attending their own group and by individual supervision with an experienced group analyst.

- *Keyworker sessions*: each PIPE resident is allocated a keyworker with whom they meet regularly, usually once each fortnight for an hour. In prisons the keyworker is also the personal officer. Keyworking supports the development of positive relationships between prisoners and staff and provides the opportunity to consider the experience of participation in the PIPE regime, as well as identifying goals and pathway planning for progression and transition through the system. Within Preparation and Provision PIPEs, keyworking will also provide the opportunity to collaboratively develop a formulation of the offender's key difficulties, usually with the input of an allocated clinician.

- *Socially creative activities*: these are informal activities, developed using a Good Lives approach, which provide prisoners and staff the opportunity to engage in a shared experience that promotes relational engagement and development. The activities may be prisoner led and provide a vehicle for authentic service user involvement.

- *Structured sessions*: these offer a formal opportunity for PIPE residents and staff to interact in a group setting. They are regular, timetabled, and tailored to each PIPE environment. Structured sessions provide an opportunity to enhance or revisit previous learning and to share experiences. In a prison setting these sessions are a mandatory requirement; however, in Approved Premises they are not compulsory, although residents are encouraged to participate, particularly when first arriving in the hostel.

While all PIPEs share the core components outlined above, the different types of PIPEs within secure settings serve different offender groups, as illustrated in Table 5.1.

The evidence base for PIPEs and their impact on psychological well-being, risk, and associated intermediate outcomes is currently very limited. An early pilot study used qualitative methods to examine the key enabling features of PIPEs in two prison services and an Approved Premise [22]. Staff, prisoners, and residents emphasized the importance of establishing and maintaining safe and supportive relationships. This included staff being available, both informally and in PIPE activities, and respectful communication and interactions.

Table 5.1 PIPE descriptions

PIPE	Population served
Preparation PIPE	Offenders who are not yet ready to engage in treatment; are unable to engage with their sentence plans; are unable to settle or progress on normal location; frequently imprisonment for public protection (IPP) or life-sentenced prisoners who are past parole.
Provision PIPE	Prisoners who are ready to engage in treatment—either accredited offending behaviour programmes or treatment for psychological and emotional difficulties—and who will benefit from the additional support provided by residing within the PIPE environment; a provision PIPE may also admit prisoners who require a period of additional support in order to achieve treatment readiness.
Progression PIPE	Admissions will usually have completed sentence plans and have no outstanding treatment needs; individuals who have completed an intensive treatment programme and require a supportive environment in which to consolidate gains made; individuals who are preparing for progression and resettlement in the community.

A consistent approach from a fully staffed team, who receive training and supervision together, was seen as central to PIPE delivery, as was the key role of the clinical lead in staff development and support. Relationships between residents or prisoners were felt to be better and, in particular, less hierarchical than in comparable non-PIPE units. Self-contained environments helped prisoners to form a more cohesive group and this could be undermined by residing in units with non-PIPE prisoners or 'lodgers'. Informal places for interaction, structured groups, creative sessions, and keywork sessions were all seen as key in supporting prosocial interactions. Support for the PIPE from the whole establishment, including frontline staff and the leadership team, was seen as important in addressing the potential of non-PIPE staff to undermine the PIPE ethos or processes.

In terms of emerging impacts, staff and prisoners/residents suggested that relationships between prisoners/residents and between staff and prisoners/residents were of a better quality. Prisoners/residents were seen to take more responsibility for their actions and behaviour and acknowledged the role of positive reinforcement from PIPE staff in maintaining treatment gains.

Ongoing evaluation of PIPEs includes a qualitative, longitudinal study of changes in social climate; the impact of a specialist training package on staff confidence and ability; a qualitative exploration of staff and prisoners'/residents' experiences of a PIPE; and an investigation of behavioural and risk changes and maintenance of change in PIPE prisoners and residents.

Enabling Environments

The Enabling Environment award, developed by the Royal College of Psychiatrists, is a quality mark that recognizes the importance of good relationships and positive and effective social environments in promoting psychological well-being [23]. Enabling Environments are defined as places:

- Where positive relationships promote well-being for all participants
- Where people experience a sense of belonging
- Where all people involved contribute to the growth and well-being of others
- Where people can learn new ways of relating
- That recognize and respect the contributions of all parties in helping relationships.

By means of a standards-based accreditation process, the award recognizes best practice in developing and maintaining healthy relational environments in a broad range of clinical and non-clinical settings. Organizations are supported to compile a portfolio of evidence that they are achieving excellence in relation to ten core standards that contribute to healthy relationships (see Table 5.2).

If an interim assessment of the evidence provided in the portfolio is successful, an assessment visit is carried out. If the organization is assessed as meeting the ten core standards of the award, the assessor makes a final report recommendation to an accreditation panel, which then ratifies the award.

While Enabling Environments are an essential component of a PIPE, they are not sufficient in themselves to be described as PIPEs, as the additional elements

Table 5.2 The ten core standards of Enabling Environments

Belonging	The nature and quality of relationships are of primary importance
Boundaries	There are expectations of behaviour and processes to maintain and review them
Communication	It is recognized that people communicate in different ways
Development	There are opportunities to be spontaneous and try new things
Involvement	Everyone shares responsibility for the environment
Safety	Support is available for everyone
Structure	Engagement and purposeful activity is actively encouraged
Empowerment	Power and authority are open to discussion
Leadership	Leadership takes responsibility for the environment being enabling
Openness	External relationships are sought and valued

of keywork sessions, socially creative activities, and structured sessions are not prerequisites.

Of particular relevance to OPD services, the Enabling Environment award recognizes that the language used to describe the core principles or experiences of positive and effective environments varies between different settings and contexts. This can make joint working between agencies difficult and result in disjointed and fragmented services. The award aims to develop a core common language applicable across a broad range of settings, including health and criminal justice, in order to more easily identify these shared themes and values.

All prison-based OPD services are expected to work towards the Enabling Environment award, emphasizing the importance of the process, as well as the award itself, but also the challenges faced in achieving the award in jointly delivered services in secure settings. The impact of Enabling Environments on the primary aims of the OPD pathway remains unclear and evaluation of such a complex intervention is challenging.

Initial work has been completed in Approved Premises to establish a baseline for staff and residents in a range of areas: these include problem solving, well-being, burnout, and the social environment, as well as residents being given a task exploring their goals and plans. Semi structured interviews are therefore undertaken before and after the Enabling Environment award is obtained [24]. Routinely collected data on recall, reconviction, and length of stay are also being collated. These data will provide a reliable benchmark against which to track future changes in Approved Premises, once they have achieved the Enabling Environment award. Baseline data are now being collected in prison, secure hospital, and housing settings where these services are also working towards the award.

Why we chose our direction

Theoretical model

The same theoretical model underpins each of the secure services developed by the LPP and is the same model on which the community services are based (see Chapter 1). It was important that the model informed a clear, consistent, and whole-team approach, while being sufficiently flexible to be applied in a range of secure settings, with different offender groups at different stages of their sentence. It was also crucial that the secure services used the same model as the community services, in order to achieve a consistent approach along the entire pathway to the community. This was achieved by using the same evidence bases, together with the same core tasks, but by adapting the means by which these tasks were worked towards, depending on the stage in the pathway and the restrictions imposed by the secure setting.

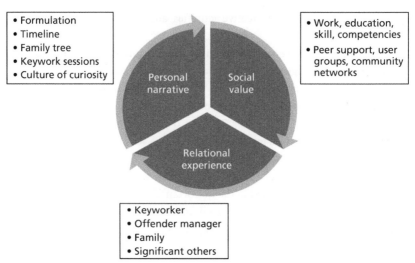

Fig. 5.1 Implementation of three core tasks of the theoretical model in secure settings

The core tasks, derived from the theoretical model, were enhancing relational experiences; increasing social value; and developing a personal narrative around the process of change, which gave meaning to the events, choices, and consequences of a non-offending way of life. The staffing, structure, mode of delivery, and intervention options were then developed with the aim of working towards these three core tasks in the context of a secure setting (see Fig. 5.1).

Operational model

Although the commissioning approach was to specify what was required for each of the three prison services out to contract, there were opportunities to shape the service in collaboration with commissioners. Our aim was to consider the service needs in terms of a matrix: the service model in relation to the intensity of intervention (see Table 5.3).

The operational model was designed to meet the needs of a diverse range of personality disordered offenders, delivered in three different prisons, and constrained by a number of factors. All three services were commissioned based on a detailed service specification which defined the target population of offenders; the catchment area; the physical location; and the aims, objectives, and outcomes of the service. Target offender populations were defined by age, sentence type, stage in sentence, and home probation location. The physical location of the services was dictated by the availability of an appropriate environment and supportive management team, which in turn defined whether or not the service would be residential, day programme, or outreach, or whether more than

Table 5.3 Considering the service model in relation to intensity of intervention

	Low intensity	Moderate intensity	High intensity
Residential programme	Core PIPE activities with the aim to settle or consolidate behaviour	Additional psychoeducational group work with the aim to develop distress tolerance and coping within a group	Additional engagement in evidence-based multi-modal therapy for personality disorder
Day programme	Drop-in and/or scheduled social and creative activities with the aim of commencing engagement	Additional psychoeducational group work with the aim to develop knowledge and skills to manage better on the wing	Additional engagement in evidence-based multi-modal therapy for personality disorder (at least twice per week)
Outreach	Attendance at complex needs planning meetings with the aim of agreeing shared formulation and engagement plan	Additional weekly contact with prisoner and with prison wing with the aim of embedding the behaviour plan and engaging the prisoner	Multiple contacts with prisoner per week by the team with the aim of progressing out of segregation or in-patient care and establishing sufficient stability to manage on the wing

one service would be delivered concurrently in the same location. The service specifications also detailed the relevant funding allocation. However, there was a degree of flexibility regarding the way in which the service specification was delivered, which allowed a more bottom-up approach to commissioning than had been the case with the DSPD services.

The operational model had to meet the needs of offenders who had never engaged in treatment previously; those who were ready for treatment; those who had already completed treatment; and those not suitable for treatment and for whom psychologically informed management was appropriate. This necessitated both treatment services and PIPEs for offenders with a wide range of previous interventions, including none, and widely varying readiness to engage. The model had to accommodate young offenders; those with both determinate and indeterminate sentences; and those approaching release to the community.

Directed by the commissioning framework and service specifications, the LPP was commissioned to deliver five services in three prisons to meet these needs (see Table 5.4).

Table 5.4 Outline of the LPP's commissioned prison services

Prison	Service
A	Category B adult male residential: low-intensity post-treatment consolidation (sixty beds); moderate-intensity pre-treatment engagement (thirty beds); high-intensity treatment provision (thirty beds). Moderate-intensity outreach
B	Category B/C adult male residential for Londoners likely to be released within two years: moderate-intensity progression (forty two beds)
C	Young adult male prison: day programme plus outreach (moderate intensity)

How to do it

Development phase

What we did

It is crucial that the joint working starts from the beginning of the development phase of the service. This provides an opportunity for staff to build a collaborative relationship; to ensure the service model is informed by a broad range of clinical and operational expertise; and to develop a sense of investment in the service that persists through to the delivery phase. OPD services challenge traditional prison culture in many ways, such that staff are continually exposed to the tension between working therapeutically and maintaining discipline. A focus on service user involvement, in particular, challenges the hierarchical structure of prison culture, and this aspect needs to be sensitively approached, as discussed in Chapter 6.

Developing a staffing structure and planning recruitment is a key early task during the development phase. In most cases, the operational lead for the service was identified by the prison service partner during the specification process and a clinical lead was tentatively identified during the bidding process. This ensured that there was strong leadership from the beginning of the development phase and that a jointly delivered ethos was evident from the start of the service delivery. Involvement of both prison and health partners in the recruitment process, both to prison officer and clinical staff posts, was generally experienced as more successful than either one partner undertaking this alone. Where possible we adopted a policy of split posts, with an element of the work in the community, which promoted continuity within the pathway.

There was inevitably limited flexibility in the choice of location for the services. However, it was important to ensure the availability of group rooms, office space, and computer access. It can be difficult to predict requirements as services develop and grow, and lack of suitable space can become a major impediment to effective service delivery. The availability of informal space is important in developing an Enabling Environment for staff and prisoners and is a key element in normalizing interactions and supporting the development of adaptive and prosocial behaviours.

Particularly if the service is to be developed in a wing that currently serves another function, and where there is going to be a period of crossover, it is important to communicate in good time with prisoners who are likely to be affected by implementation of the service, including those who currently reside on the wing identified for service development.

Wherever possible, training was delivered jointly to both clinical and prison staff. The broader approach to training is discussed in Chapter 2. However, in the secure services, emphasis was placed on what clinical and operational staff could learn from each other. Training also had to be adapted to fit in with the prison regime and to maximize attendance of prison staff who worked shifts. Aligning training with the wider prison staff training days and delivering regular, brief sessions where shifts overlapped were particularly helpful.

Another key early task is to ensure that there is the understanding and support from the governing governor and senior management team. This can be achieved through informal discussions, presentations to senior prison staff outlining the service model, and consultation over the impact of the service on the wider establishment. Communication about the service also needs to filter through all levels of operation within an establishment, to ensure that service is supported both by those working in it and throughout frontline staff. Raising awareness and providing training for the wider establishment including operational staff and other departments within the prison is also helpful. In particular, it is essential to make a particular effort to liaise and form good working relationships with departments within the prison likely to interface with the service, such as healthcare, the offender management unit (OMU), segregation, and substance-use services.

What we learned

Although all three OPD prison services were based on the same theoretical model, they have all developed significantly in response to the emerging demands and constraints posed by their particular prisoner groups and environments. Nevertheless, our consortium model has allowed rapid dissemination of good practice between the three services, as well as shared learning when each has encountered difficulties, and avoided the feeling of isolation which is common amongst specialist services in secure environments.

The joint commissioning of the services has been one of the clearest successes of the delivery of the OPD pathway in secure settings. Relationships between commissioners and providers have been good and have remained so from the development phase through to the delivery of the established services. There has been a strong sense of collaboration in ensuring the success of the services, balancing the flexibility needed in piloting complex services with robust scrutiny of performance indicators. The commissioners have also been invaluable in managing the relationship between health and criminal justice providers, which has, on occasion, been less straightforward. For example, where prisons have to prioritize security, this can threaten the stability of a developing service, as staff are cross-deployed to perform core duties elsewhere. Conversely, there can be a tendency for operational staff to defer to the perceived expertise of the health provider, leading to partnership imbalance.

Liaison with the rest of the prison has ensured that areas of possible replication or conflict can be identified and addressed. Suspicion of and resentment towards OPD services are perhaps to be anticipated, and certainly prison officers on the OPD units have received some negative feedback from peers for the ways in which they carry out their new role. Historically, 'health' services have often been experienced as experts imposing their ways of working in a system that they do not fully understand and which they expect to adapt to them. There is also significant overlap between the function of the OPD services and other departments with the prisons, particularly the OMUs, psychology, and mental health in-reach teams. Establishing good relationships with the OMUs has been crucial in managing referrals into the units and both transfers out and releases.

Supervision and reflective practice were invariably viewed with suspicion to begin with and then embraced by both prison officers and clinical staff. Prison officers often felt that reflective practice was self-indulgent and that supervision was covert psychological assessment. Clinical staff often felt more inhibited in reflective practice with prison officers than they might in a more conventional clinical setting, in case they might be seen as either emotionally vulnerable or showing off. In all services, all staff came to value both reflective practice and supervision as being key to maintaining a psychologically informed approach to their work in the services.

Difficulties arising from the prison regime were not prominent in the LPP prison services. However, one or two operational issues were a persistent cause for concern for both prisoners and staff. Particularly when the services were new and had yet to reach full occupancy, 'lodgers' from other parts of the prison were frequently transferred into vacant cells in the residential services. Often these were prisoners who had created management difficulties on other wings in the prison, and transfers were most common at night and weekends. Prisoners on the LPP services often felt that these lodgers undermined the sense of community and containment in the service and, particularly if they remained on the unit for some time, could cause problems due to intimidation and bullying.

Referral and assessment

What we did

Our principle was that we should deliver accessible services—that is, services which were responsive to referrals, not overly demanding, and which tried to adapt interventions to meet the needs of the referred population. We therefore did not insert obstacles into the process, such as onerous referral processes or drawn-out assessment periods. Written information detailing the service plan and admission criteria was provided to the referrer and prisoner prior to assessment.

Assessments were jointly undertaken by clinical and operational staff and, ideally, in person. However, because potential prisoners could have been in any prison in England, a practical alternative is assessment by video link. Given that it is largely possible to establish whether or not the prisoner meets the admission criteria for the service prior to assessment, the key tasks of the meeting are to (1) provide information about the service; (2) assess the prisoner's motivation to engage; (3) review the prisoner's recent behaviour; and (4) get the prisoner's perspective on their risk, needs, and where they have had difficulties.

No psychometric assessment is necessary and it is helpful to emphasize that a diagnosis of personality disorder is not necessary either to be eligible for the service or to benefit from it. Concerns about the specific prison the service is located in should be addressed and it should be emphasized that the services are not mental health services and that they are part of a pathway of services, including those in the community. While it is important to emphasize the benefits of the service, including the environment, if appropriate, it is important not to oversell the service and to point out difficulties that may be encountered in making the decision to engage and to change. At the end of the assessment, prisoners should be informed about the decision-making process, the timing of this, and how it will be communicated to them. Assessments should be then discussed with the team and a joint decision regarding appropriateness for admission made. Consideration should be given to the timing of the assessment. It is often best to leave assessments until after pending Parole Board hearings so that prisoners do not feel pressured into agreeing to engage in order to make a favourable impression. It is also to be expected that it may take more than one assessment before a prisoner decides that the service might be helpful for him or her, and follow-up arrangements should be made in such cases. If the prisoner is assessed as suitable, it is important to obtain relevant security or intelligence information, so that appropriate assessments can be made of potential risks specific to the proposed service. It has also been helpful to arrange an agreement for the referring prison to accept the prisoner back within six months of transfer if the prisoner is deselected. This avoids deselected prisoners remaining in the service and potentially being disruptive, but also reassures potential prisoners that they will not be 'trapped' in the service if they subsequently feel they have made the wrong decision in transferring there.

What we learned

One of the key advantages of joint working that became evident from early on in the delivery of the services was the impact on engaging prisoners. Many prisoners who had never previously been able to engage in offending behaviour work and who had caused significant management problems responded positively to attempts to engage them in OPD services. While the novelty of the services piqued the interest of some and the additional resources, both in terms of staff and the environment, were undoubtedly helpful, the joint approach appeared to allow them to overcome their reservations about both the health and criminal justice systems. The services did not quite carry the stigma associated with mental health services and the lack of the need for any diagnosis and the management or coaching, rather than treatment, approach seemed to appeal to those who had either never accessed mental health services before or had difficult experiences when they did. At the same time, the embedding of psychology staff in the prison allowed for engagement strategies tailored to the individual's personality difficulties and for a 'slow-burn', low-key approach, rather than an all-or-nothing one-off assessment. The fact that the referral was supported by everyone involved in the prisoner's management also seemed to reduce the anxiety that differences in opinion in relation to the suggested pathway would result in yet more, conflicting recommendations once they completed the work proposed in the OPD services. The culture of curiosity in the services and the emphasis placed on addressing problems in the interpersonal context of day-to-day life on the unit also helped ensure that engagement was maintained and that drop-outs or deselection were minimized.

Interventions

What we did

The development of the treatment programme was influenced by a number of factors related to the theoretical model underpinning the services; the characteristics of the prisoner group; and the constraints of the prison regime and environment. It was important that the interventions were evidence informed, particularly by the attachment and desistance literature, and that they were delivered in an interpersonal or group context. While factors common to most treatment approaches to personality disorder were adopted, such as structure, consistency, and an emphasis on the treatment alliance, it was recognized that some specific models are better at targeting specific domains of personality pathology. This is in keeping with Livesley's integrated modular approach to the treatment of personality disorder [25].

In terms of the prisoner group, it was important to take into account the fact that many of the prisoners had never engaged in either offending behaviour programmes or psychological treatment previously. At the same time, others had completed years of treatment and there was a risk of simply replicating what they had already done. Therefore, the overall programme had to be sufficiently flexible to provide individual programmes of appropriate intensity. Although all prisoners had personality difficulties, these were diverse, and this too had to be recognized in the development of the treatment programme.

Group work had to fit in with the prison regime, in terms of both availability of staff and avoiding clashes with other activities and tasks prisoners had to undertake in the limited time they were unlocked from their cells. It was also helpful to have components of treatment that could be jointly delivered by clinical and operational staff and that had some continuity with the treatment available in the community.

Although the treatment programmes varied between the different services depending on the age of the prisoners, whether the service was residential or a day programme, and the stage the prisoners were at in their pathway, they all had two main goals—that is, to assist offenders in developing a personal narrative about their lives and their difficulties (past, present, and future) and to help them think about relational issues by means of participation in a group-related activity. Although the aims remained the same, the intensity and degree of sophistication of the interventions differed between prisoners, depending on their needs and responsivity factors. In addition to informal interaction between staff and prisoners, every prisoner had to agree, as a minimum, to engage in jointly delivered keywork, with the aim of addressing intervention planning, formulation, family tree, desistance plan, and relapse triggers. Psychoeducation and skills groups comprised the next level of intensity. Psychoeducation groups tended to be no more than four sessions long and focused on themes such as understanding personality difficulties and knowing your own risk. Skills groups were of a similar duration and focused on managing difficulties such as anger and paranoia. The highest-level intensity interventions were longer duration, mixed modal treatment based on evidence-informed approaches, such as mentalization-based treatment, schema-focused therapy, and dialectical behaviour therapy. All groups were delivered as part of a rolling programme, so that there were multiple opportunities for prisoners to access each group at various stages in their time on the unit. The flexible, modular approach meant that individual programmes could be devised that were of an appropriate intensity and which took into consideration the prisoner's specific personality difficulties and any treatment completed previously.

What we learned

Keywork sessions were valued by both prisoners and staff. Prisoners reported that the relationship they developed with their keyworker changed their attitude towards authority and gave them the optimism and understanding needed to change. Giving some consideration to keyworker allocation following assessment of prisoners seemed to be a worthwhile task. Prison officers often reported feeling anxious or deskilled initially when providing keywork sessions (or displayed varying degrees of avoidance). However, most came to value the relationship with their keyworkers as the positive impact of what was often experienced as a difficult process became evident. Very few conflicts between prisoners and their keyworkers were not ultimately resolved and most requests to change, from both sides, were withdrawn or not maintained when additional support was provided.

Another important aspect of the service model was the emphasis on developing a shared understanding of the prisoner's difficulties, risk, and needs. Many prisoners reported either disengaging from services or pseudo-engaging with them in the past, as they did not recognize the way in which their problems had been conceptualized to them. Having the flexibility to frame difficulties using a range of different language and theoretical approaches meant that common ground could almost always be achieved and any understanding did not feel imposed on the prisoner. This, in turn, often formed a foundation from which the prisoner felt more disposed to persevere with other formulations introduced in the context of further work, which they might previously have rejected outright.

Good working relationships with mental health in-reach teams and with psychology were also key to the success of the services. Discussion in the development stages of the services ensured that the remit of both services was mutually understood, and regular meetings allowed for flexibility such that mental health in-reach staff continued to work with patients with personality disorder with whom they had established a productive therapeutic relationship. Similarly, responsibility for the management of comorbid mental illness could be discussed on a case by case basis, while maintaining clear clinical governance arrangements.

Pathway progression

What we did

Ensuring progression on the OPD pathway was one of the key tasks of all the secure services, whether this was progression into treatment in a secure service or progression from custody into the community pathway. A systematic approach to monitoring progression while in the services was underpinned by regular keywork sessions, where interventions could be planned in a sequential way and key goals defined and reviewed. Working with the community offender manager and arranging regular three-way meetings in the prison was instrumental in promoting progression. Where heavy offender manager workloads made more regular contact unrealistic, meetings planned to coincide with anticipated milestones or transitions such as Parole Board hearings or release were prioritized. Staff also formally reviewed each prisoner's progress by liaising with their offender supervisor, participating in relevant Multi-Agency Public Protection Arrangements (MAPPA) and by providing written and oral evidence to the Parole Board.

For those being released, prisoners reviewed their desistance plans with their keyworker in anticipation of release and put together plans for their first week following release, with particular focus on the first forty eight hours. These, together with the prisoner's formulation, would be shared with professionals involved in their supervision and care, so that they could continue to be refined as the offender progressed along the pathway. Prisoners are given an electronic travel card and a basic mobile phone on release and are taken through the gate by their keyworker, who accompanies them to their first appointment, generally with their offender manager or Approved Premises worker. Staff from the secure service follow the offender up in the first week post-release and again at an agreed later date. A voicemail service is also provided, so that offenders can contact the unit if they encounter any difficulties, with the expectation that they will be contacted by the staff the same day.

For prisoners whose next progressive move is anticipated to be to another secure service, staff help the prisoner identify the service most appropriate to meet their needs and support the referral and assessment process. This is particularly straightforward if the service is another LPP service. However, the process is also enhanced by developing good relationships with other secure services in the OPD pathway, often by the process of making a first referral to the service but also through various OPD network meetings.

What we learned

Working collaboratively in sentence planning ensured that progress made in the services informed sentence plans and that treatment plans addressed outstanding sentence targets. It provided an opportunity for innovative approaches to pathway planning, informed by an understanding of risk, personality difficulties, and pathway options. It also ensured that both written and oral evidence of this progress was made available to the Parole Board. One issue that had to be addressed early on, both with OMUs and psychology, was the practice of health professionals who delivered treatment to an individual commenting on both the treatment and risk, as well as making recommendations to the Parole Board. The apparent conflict in doing so, well recognized within the criminal justice system, was subsequently addressed by health staff providing treatment reports and pathway options, without commenting on risk or making specific recommendations. This felt counter to health staff's instincts, not least because they had been treating and risk-assessing individuals for years in health settings, but also because the initial reports were often enthusiastically welcomed by the Parole Board. Teething problems with the Parole Board included the need to separate the tasks of risk assessment and treatment, such that they were not provided by, and reported on, by the same individual, and the tendency for any new service to be seen as a prerequisite for release for anyone with a personality disorder, whether or not he or she requires it or is willing to participate. These difficulties improved considerably following a series of successful open days in the services, specifically for members of the Parole Board.

The provision of both community and secure OPD services by a single consortium was a considerable advantage in developing pathways through OPD services. Each secure service and the community services could adapt to developing needs and ensure as smooth transitions as possible. Systematic case identification and the fact that several staff worked across both secure and community settings ensured awareness was maintained amongst offender managers in the community and a consistent number of high-quality referrals. In the same way, through OPD prison service network meetings and contact through referrals and visits from other prison OPD services, a number of pathways into and out of each unit were established. Continuity of both staff and model 'through the gate' and detailed release plans also supported the risk management of this high-risk period. However, despite this, longstanding difficulties, such as lack of appropriate accommodation and specialist forensic personality disorder services in the community, continued to limit the success of desistance and release planning.

Evaluation

External evaluation

An independent evaluation of the progression service used a qualitative approach and psychometric assessment to assess the impact of the service on offenders' understanding of their risk and the strategies needed to manage them [26]. The evaluation also examined the factors associated with engagement in the service and the processes underpinning any change seen as a result.

Prisoners demonstrated a good understanding of their risk factors for reoffending and why these factors were related to their risk. They were also generally realistic about obstacles to desistance from offending and emphasized the importance of support following release in overcoming these. Prisoners and staff were in broad agreement about what changed as a result of being in the service and how. Prisoners changed their attitude towards authority, improved their understanding of themselves, and gained a greater sense of self-worth and optimism through the positive relationships developed with staff during keywork sessions. They learned new skills in the context of course work, but also by facing up to difficulties on the wing. Prisoners and staff agreed on the obstacles to change, which were largely due to the security restrictions associated with the service being located in a high-secure prison. Restrictions on delivering release on temporary licence and some other activities led to prisoners feeling let down and having negative, counter-therapeutic attitudes. Prisoners reported a number of factors that hindered engagement in the programme. These included a lack of meaningful activity, a reduction in the number of keywork sessions, understaffing, and a perception that they had completed all the work they needed to do. The particular prisoner mix also had an impact on engagement, where the behaviour and needs of older indeterminate-sentenced prisoners and younger determinate-sentenced prisoners were not always compatible. However, despite motivational issues, most prisoners attended sessions, citing personal benefit, affiliation with their keyworker, and commitment to the community as the reasons for doing so.

Parallel psychometric assessment of the mechanisms underlying changes seen as a result of being in the service showed that prisoners were highly ready for change and showed some improvement in engagement over time. There was evidence of improved problem solving, with less avoidance and impulsivity, and improved emotion regulation. However, that latter finding was largely accounted for by improved awareness and there was no evidence of change in access to strategies for emotion regulation. Interestingly, there were marked changes identified in interpersonal style while in the service, with prisoners becoming more dominant, coercive, hostile, withdrawn, and submissive, and less compliant, nurturing, and gregarious. It was unclear whether or not this reflected changes towards optimum levels in each of these domains, problems with engagement, or a possible adverse impact of being in the service on some individuals.

National evaluations of the OPD pathway and of individual components of the pathway including DTCs and PIPEs have been jointly commissioned by HMPPS and NHSE and will report in the next few years.

Internal evaluation

Table 5.5 outlines the activity of the three LPP OPD pathway prison units over the first two years of operation. For the young adult offender institution, with a day centre model, there has been successful engagement with a number of high-risk antisocial individuals participating in both individual and group therapy. Although only eight individuals dropped out of treatment, a further twenty five were 'shipped out' of the prison during the course of treatment due to their involvement in ongoing violence or conflicts within the prison. Prison 2 has been overwhelmed with referrals to its sixty pre-treatment/treatment beds, largely because of the pressing need for the pre-treatment facility. Again, around one-third are deselected, but an equal number progressed on their sentence plan in a positive direction, moving on to less-secure conditions. Interestingly, although prison 3 drew from a slightly different population of offenders returning to London who were drawing nearer to the possibility of release, the picture remains fairly similar—the only difference being that of the thirty positive progressions, ten of these were automatic releases into the community for determinate-sentenced prisoners.

A number of internal evaluation projects have been commissioned by the LPP, including a qualitative study of prisoners who have failed to make progressive moves from LPP OPD prison services and an evaluation of the pathway of

Table 5.5 Throughput in the three OPD pathway prison units (2014–2016)

	Prison 1	Prison 2	Prison 3
Referrals	280	687	260
Admissions	84 (30%)	122 (18%)	81 (31%)
De-selections	33 (39%)	36 (30%)	30 (37%)
Positive sentence progression	11 (13%)	35 (29%)	20 (25%) + 10
Currently in service	40	56	21

prisoners who have been recalled to prison having previously been in a prison OPD service.

Next steps

The secure services described in this chapter are in a continuous process of consolidating what has been found to be effective and developing in response to what has been found not to work as well as expected. This will continue over the next phase of these services. However, the focus will shift slightly to responding to the national evaluation of the OPD pathway, which will report in 2018, and the development of a more extensive internal research and service improvement programme. The latter will aim to examine points across the pathway in London where progression is slow or can be blocked, and to evaluate those offenders who fail to make progressive moves and whose needs may not be being met by the pathway in its current form.

The services will have to respond to the commissioning environment, including anticipated contract reviews and tendering timeframes, but also potential developments in the pathway, such as services for specific groups of personality disordered offenders, including those with comorbid neurodevelopmental disorders and those who have committed sex offences. The LPP will work with commissioners to identify changes in need on a local level and to refine existing services and develop new ones where gaps are identified, including the development of OPD services in open prison conditions.

References

1. **Lipton DS, Pearson FS, Cleland CM, Yee D.** The effectiveness of cognitive-behavioural treatment methods on recidivism. In J McGuire (Ed.), Offender rehabilitation and treatment: effective programmes and policies to reduce re-offending. Chichester: John Wiley & Sons; 2002, pp. 79–112.

2. **McGuire J.** What works to reduce reoffending: 18 years on. In LA Craig, L Dixon, and TA Gannon (Eds.), What works in offender rehabilitation: an evidence based approach to assessment and treatment. Chichester: Wiley-Blackwell; 2013, pp. 20–49.

3. **Andrews DA, Bonta J, Hoge RD.** Classification for effective rehabilitation: rediscovering psychology. Criminal Justice and Behaviour. 1990;**17**:19–52.

4. **Friendship C, Blud L, Erikson M, Travers R, Thornton D.** Cognitive-behavioural treatment for imprisoned offenders: an evaluation of HM Prison Service's cognitive skills programmes. Legal and Criminological Psychology. 2003;**8**:103–114.

5. **Andrews DA, Bonta J.** The psychology of criminal conduct, 4th edn. Newark, NJ: LexisNexis; 2006.

6. **Home Office.** The impact of corrections on re-offending: a review of 'what works'. London: Home Office; 2005.

7. **Warren F, Preedy-Fayers K, McGauley G,** et al. Review of treatments for severe personality disorder. Home Office Online Report 30/30. London: Home Office; 2003. http://citeseerx.ist.psu.edu/viewdoc/download?doi=10.1.1.614.6986&rep=rep1&type=pdf.

8. **McMurran M, Hubard N, Duggan C.** A comparison of treatment completers and non-completers of an in-patient treatment programme for male personality-disordered offenders. Psychology and Psychotherapy: Theory, Research and Practice. 2008;**81**(2):193–198.

9. **McMuran M, Hubbard N, Overton E.** Non-completion of personality disorder treatments: a systematic review of correlates, consequences, and interventions. Clinical Psychology Review. 2010;**30**(3):277–287.

10. **Chiesa M, Fonagy P.** Cassel personality disorder study: methodology and treatment effects. British Journal of Psychiatry. 2000;**176**:485–491.

11. **Lees A, Manning N, Rawlings B.** A culture of enquiry: research evidence and the therapeutic community. Psychiatric Quarterly. 2004;**75**(3):279–294.

12. **Newberry M.** A synthesis of outcome research at Grendon Therapeutic Community Prison. Therapeutic Communities. 2010;**31**(4):356–371.

13. **Tew J, Atkinson R.** The Chromis programme: from conception to evaluation. Psychology, Crime & Law. 2013;**19**:415–431.

14. **Fallon P, Bluglass R, Edwards B, Daniels G.** Report of the Committee of Inquiry into the Personality Disorder Unit, Ashworth Special Hospital. London: The Stationery Office; 1994.

15. **Sparr LF.** Personality disorders and criminal law: an international perspective. Journal of the American Academy of Psychiatry and the Law. 2009;**37**:168–181.

16. **Beyer AD, Cheung M.** Sexually violent predators and civil commitment laws. Journal of Child Sexual Abuse. 2004;**13**(2):41–57.

17. **Trestman RL, Eucker S, Muller-Isberner R.** The treatment of personality-disordered offenders in Germany. Journal of the American Academy of Psychiatry and the Law. 2007;**35**:229–234.

18. **Kersten L, Cislo AM, Lynch M, Shea K, Trestman RL.** Evaluating START NOW: a skills-based psychotherapy for inmates of correctional systems. Psychiatric Services. 2016;**67**:37–42.

19. **Ministry of Justice, Department of Health.** A guide to Psychologically Informed Planned Environments (PIPEs). Version 1. London: Department of Health; 2012.

20. **Turner K, Bolger L.** The provision of PIPEs—Psychologically Informed Planned Environments. Prison Service Journal. 2015;**218**:41–46.

21. **Brown M.** Psychologically Informed Planned Environment—PIPE: a group analytic perspective. Psychoanalytic Psychotherapy. 2014;**28**:345–354.

22. **Turley C.** Enabling features of psychologically informed planned environments. London: NatCen Social Research, Ministry of Justice Analytical Services; 2013.

23. **Royal College of Psychiatrists.** Enabling Environment standards. London: Royal College of Psychiatrists; 2013.

24. **Davies J, O'Meara A.** Routine practice in staffed community accommodation (approved premises) in England and Wales: quantitative benchmarking from the first year of a longitudinal study. Criminal Behaviour and Mental Health. 2018;**28**:227–238.

25. **Livesley WJ, Clarkin JF.** A general framework for integrated modular treatment. In WJ Livesley, G Dimaggio, and JF Clarkin (Eds.), Integrated treatment for personality disorder: a modular approach. New York: Guilford Press; 2016.

26. **McMurran M, Delight S.** Process of change in an offender personality disorder pathway prison progression unit. Criminal Behaviour and Mental Health. 2017;27:254–264.

Chapter 6

Meaningful service user participation in the pathway

Nikki Jeffcote, Karen Van Gerko, and Emma Nicklin

Introduction

In recent years there has been a fundamental change in the relationship between service users and professionals across the western world, with the notion of 'user participation' becoming central to service design and delivery. The concept of working in collaboration and partnership with users of health services has become embedded in the design and delivery of those services, as well as in professionals' training and continuing professional development. In the UK public sector this movement has been the result of a number of factors:

- Widespread social, technological, and economic change: increased access to and dissemination of information of all kinds through the internet has altered the balance of power between organizations, agencies providing services, and the people who use those services. In the general health arena, this has led to a reorientation of the user–provider relationship, with increased focus on informed consent, choice, and user feedback, and to the development of a more personalized, collaborative, and shared approach to the management of health conditions.

- A recognition of the many and diverse stakeholders in any public service: increasingly, a '360-degree' approach informs the evolution and development of services. In addition to policymakers, commissioners, and providers, the involvement of service users, carers, and staff, together with non-statutory organizations, local communities, and special interest groups, is regarded as essential to effective outcomes. For example, the Sainsbury Centre for Mental Health [1] recommends that peer professionals should make up half the workforce in mental health services, to ensure recovery approaches are made a reality.

- The development of non-statutory services led by users and former users of services: there has been significant growth in user-led organizations, which may provide information to users and feedback to service providers, campaign for change, and offer mutual validation and support. Within mental health, there is recognition of the valuable role of peer support in promoting recovery, validating user experience, and enabling users' voices to be heard where they can make a difference. These approaches are now supported by current UK government policy [2].

- A culture that values individual agency and control, and responds to the democratic power of collective concerns: society has become increasingly reflexive and aware as the precedents set by previous social structures and traditions have reduced in their influence [3]. Since the 1990s this has been reflected in the Department of Health's increasing commitment to the notion that individuals with personal experience of mental health problems can directly effect change across the planning and delivery of care [4]. This is reflected in the key principles of personalization and choice, as well as the social inclusion agenda.

- A recognition that services are enhanced by diversity amongst service providers: in a complex and multi-cultural society there is a multiplicity of individual experiences and narratives. Diversity amongst those delivering as well as receiving a service validates service users' perspectives and identities, potentially enhancing engagement and well-being.

- A recognition that in a post-recession world, contributions that are not resource- or expertise-intensive have a key role to play in sustainable services: efficiency involves ensuring that each aspect of a service is provided by the people who are best suited to deliver it. For certain kinds of support, service user peers may be the most appropriate facilitators, for example in reducing isolation and helping someone to ask the right questions. Enabling individuals to direct their own care has been shown to contribute to reducing the demands on services [5].

User groups are increasingly integrated into service provision at all levels [6]; however, for offenders who have significant social, health, and criminogenic needs, the picture is more complicated. In the UK, the concept of the offender as a 'service user' with whom social-work-trained professionals built a collaborative working relationship was supplanted in the 1990s when the role of 'probation officer' was recast as the 'offender manager', whose job was to supervise rather than support. A procedural rather than relational approach to risk management developed, with an increased reliance on restrictive approaches that were seen as defensible but had the potential to exacerbate some risk factors, particularly social isolation. In custodial settings, the need to maintain control and discipline, and to protect both staff and prisoners from the potential consequences of high levels of negative emotion, has led to an approach that focuses primarily on behavioural management and procedural and physical security. This has unwittingly diverted attention away from considering individual prisoners' states of mind. As a result, the notion of working in partnership with offenders can be perceived as threatening across the criminal justice system. In this mindset, collaboration is viewed as increasing rather than mitigating risk, reflecting a loss of skills and confidence in managing boundaries relationally and a reliance on defensive risk management strategies.

In this chapter we describe our approach to involving our service users in both prison and community service development. These are men and women at high risk of violent and/or sexual reoffending, who have significant personality difficulties that are linked to their risk. This is still 'work in progress' and service users are not yet truly embedded as partners in the services we provide, but we have learned much over the last four years and aim to share some of our experience to support others on a similar journey. In the sections that follow, we describe the journey from our perspective as providers, and include service users' accounts of their experience of that journey.

We begin by reviewing the literature on user involvement in forensic services, then outline the available models of user involvement, before describing the choices we made. We go on to illustrate our practice with examples from the community, and service users from the LPP service user forum have made a significant contribution to this section of the chapter. We then conclude with reflections on our progress and possible next steps.

Literature review

Theoretical background

In recent years, health service users have increasingly sought and gained empowerment to bring about positive changes in services. The recovery movement and personalization approaches to mental health involve choice and control, and the concept of 'co-production' has gained increasing currency. Nevertheless, challenges remain in moving beyond tokenism to genuine partnership and influence.

Theorists of meaningful user involvement have tended to focus on process issues rather than outcomes, and on the centrality of communicative processes. Davies and colleagues [7] observed that 'service user involvement is not an end in itself, but a means of effecting change, both in the outcomes of services and the behaviours of workers'.

User involvement operates at many levels. At its most simple, it is about the service user actively participating in shaping the service and support he/she receives. More widely, it means actively including service user perspectives in the design, commissioning, delivery, and evaluation of services and in policy development. NHS England [8] commissioned a programme in which patient leadership was explored with a view to identifying good practice across health organizations. The programme recommended investing in patient leaders to influence service priorities and design, so that patient care remains at the heart of delivery, and establishing a commitment to qualitative feedback processes through the development of cultures and systems that ensure organizations listen.

There are various ways in which this process can be thought about. An early concept was the 'ladder of participation' [9], developed to encompass different ideas about possible 'levels' of involvement. These might include provision of information (the lowest level of participation); consultation with users; active participation through making suggestions and influencing outcomes; sharing decisions and responsibility; and on to full ownership, where users control decision making at the highest level. As described in Chapter 1, the Offender Personality Disorder (OPD) pathway programme adopts a 'whole system approach' and services are encouraged to attend to four aspects of embedded user involvement:

- Structure: whereby the planning, development and resourcing of user involvement are evident in the organization's structure
- Review: having systems in place to monitor and evaluate changes brought about by involving service users
- Practice: incorporating ways of working that include the involvement of service users in day-to-day practice and processes
- Culture: creating an organizational ethos in which user involvement is an accepted element of the service and is recognized by both staff and service users as integral to its aims and operation.

As well as drawing on frameworks such as these, service user involvement initiatives need to be transparent and reflective about issues of power. An Australian study by Byrne et al. [10] explored the experiences of 'lived experience practitioners' in mental health services. They found that the dominance of the medical model imposed significant limitations on the implementation, effectiveness, and development of these practitioner roles; the medical model was perceived by them as obstructing recovery. Essentially, power depends on a range of things: information, money, skills, confidence, and vested authority. It is also inherently relational and is often implicitly thought of as binary—you have it or you don't. This is likely to be particularly the case in services for personality disordered offenders, whose own experiences of abuse and antisocial subcultures have frequently created in their minds a strongly hierarchical internal model of relationships, in which the primary available positions are dominance and submission. These internal models are themselves powerful and can become enacted in the wider system. The structures of criminal justice systems, and the real power of professionals to make decisions that have profound impacts on users' lives, in any case tend to reinforce this model of relating. The result is a reified understanding of power as quantitative—there is only so much to go round. Meaningful participation means being realistic about imbalances in external power and control, while recognizing the potential for empowerment to be mutual, and that working together achieves more than either side can do alone.

Key developments in service user involvement in mental health and prisons

Secure settings present specific difficulties in achieving meaningful participation and open communication. Trust between staff and service users is difficult to establish, communication is constrained by imbalances of power and authority, and there are limits on what can be talked about: not everything is up for discussion [11, 12]. Professionals always have higher status and hold more power. In mental health services, users' voices may explicitly and implicitly be silenced or undermined by assumptions that a psychiatric diagnosis invalidates a person's articulated experience. A similar process can operate with offenders, who may be viewed as having somehow forfeited their right to a voice by their crimes. The language of criminal justice systems also tends to undermine the perceived value of users' perspectives: for example, the concept of 'corrections' implies something 'wrong' with the individual that needs 'correcting'; and defining someone as an 'offender' obscures other aspects of his or her identity. Staff—both in prison and in the community—may be fearful of the risks of involving service users in service design and delivery, and have little faith in the possibility of any benefit.

Against this challenging background, some pockets of active user involvement have nevertheless developed in the criminal justice system. In prisons in the UK, one of the earliest systemic examples of user involvement was the Listeners scheme run by The Samaritans, a charity established in the 1950s to 'befriend the suicidal and despairing'. Samaritan volunteers provide support to prisoner volunteers, who offer befriending support to distressed peers. This scheme has now been embedded in prisons in England and Wales for over fifteen years. Peer mentoring is well established as a mechanism for addressing a range of needs in prison, such as literacy problems and substance misuse. More recently, user councils have been developed in some UK jails, supported by a user-led charity, User Voice, in which nominated prisoner representatives from different areas of the prison sit on a working group that has real influence and decision-making powers. The same charity has supported the development of user councils in community probation services, obtaining peer feedback and making recommendations as to how services can be improved for users. The success of these initiatives illustrates some of the key requirements of effective user involvement, which include: listening to and addressing the concerns and views of professionals and staff; identifying credible 'champions' who are able to authentically convey the potential benefits of an involvement strategy; robust risk management policies and procedures; and regular review and evaluation to establish effectiveness and identify emerging problems.

In the areas of both mental health and substance misuse—where the user populations to some extent overlap with the offending population—the mutual aid, or 'self-help', group has been developed internationally as a model of peer support. It may include the provision of treatment delivered exclusively by service users without professional input. This is not, as far as we are aware, a model that has been replicated with offenders, but it demonstrates the potential for empowerment amongst some of the most excluded members of society.

Service user involvement and 'high-risk, high-harm' personality disordered offenders

Personality disordered offenders are doubly disadvantaged. They suffer the same range of difficulties experienced by others with mental health problems and in addition experience the stigma and exclusion that accompany a history of serious offending. Many prisoners who have served lengthy sentences are released into a community in which the infrastructure of daily life has changed radically, with little or nothing by way of support or guidance to navigate this alien world. The challenges they face in attempting to develop prosocial identities and manage safer lives include the following:

- Limited positive social networks and a high degree of social isolation
- Antisocial peers, associates, and neighbours
- Difficult family relationships, often activating unhelpful relationship patterns and high levels of emotional arousal
- Lack of practical and work-related skills
- Limited access to education, employment, and voluntary opportunities that require a criminal record check

- Repeated experiences of failure in the past that impair and inhibit new learning
- Poor physical health/well-being linked to difficulties in looking after themselves
- Difficulties accessing practical and emotional support effectively, due to poor relationships with attachment and authority figures
- Coping strategies that may bring other problems in their wake (e.g. avoidance; substance misuse)
- Negative social attitudes towards them and lack of non-statutory/third-sector organizations providing relevant support
- Approaches to risk management by criminal justice and other agencies that are frequently restrictive and reinforce avoidance, leading to an increasingly impoverished way of life.

These environmental, relational, and internal obstacles highlight the scale of the challenge for high-risk personality disordered offenders in trying to build a safe life in the community. They also relate closely to the factors that have in recent years been identified as central to desistance from offending, as articulated in an extensive body of research.

Desistance is the process by which someone stops offending, and we have found the desistance literature relevant and useful in thinking about how to integrate meaningful user involvement into services. The research indicates some key elements in desistance: developing a meaningful social role; building a network of supportive and prosocial relationships; and developing a narrative of one's past life and offending that facilitates the imagination and gradual realization of a new identity as a non-offending citizen [13]. Developing a new, non-offender identity is a process crucially supported by having someone who can sustain a belief that such an identity is possible, even when the offender him- or herself is losing hope. For most service users, professionals have an important part to play in this; however, they cannot be role models in the same way as someone who has themselves already trodden the path to desistance; nor can they offer guidance on the basis of what has worked for them personally.

Challenges to desistance—including many of the factors identified above, such as financial hardship, substance misuse, and lack of housing—are acknowledged in the literature, but there has tended to be a prevailing view that, in the absence of relapse to offending, the individual will find other reinforcers and carry on to establish a crime-free identity as a non-offender [14]. In this interpretation, maintenance of desistance is seen as a relatively straightforward positive outcome for both the former offender and the wider community [15]. However, there is also evidence that desistance from offending is for some people associated with self-imposed restrictions and avoidance of risky situations, which leads to an impoverished lifestyle, reinforces low self-esteem, and perpetuates social isolation, without any positive benefits of a new, non-offender identity [16]. This has been clearly evident amongst the high-risk personality disordered individuals who use our services, many of whom are only able to envisage staying safe through isolation and withdrawal.

It is therefore increasingly recognized that interventions for high-risk offenders should aim to strengthen protective factors alongside other measures promoting external and internal controls. The evidence suggests that services should find new ways of promoting and supporting former offenders' social participation, capitalizing on their strengths and recognizing and responding to the barriers they face, and creating meaningful opportunities to live differently [17].

McNeill [18] comments, 'Desistance is a social process as much as a personal one'. The concept of 'zero tolerance' for antisocial behaviour in public services increases the potential for excluding individuals whose difficulties include poor emotional and behavioural self-management, particularly in situations of vulnerability and interactions with authority figures and caregivers. The options for promoting involvement are therefore constrained both by the nature of the users' difficulties and by barriers in the external and social environment.

Peer relationships represent both a major strength and a major challenge of the OPD pathway programme. The internal world of personality disordered offenders is often fragmented, fearful, and conflictual, and these are qualities that tend also to be found in the systems around them. Historically, attitudes to risk management of offenders in the community have tended to be restrictive, focusing on what the person is not allowed to do. This includes restrictions with respect to employment, training, education, relationships of various kinds, and, in some cases, geographical limitations. Antisocial and criminal associates are a major risk factor for reoffending, and association with other offenders is often explicitly prohibited under the terms of statutory supervision for many UK offenders with sexual convictions. Against this background, building a culture of 'positive risk taking' may often be as anxiety-provoking for service users as it is for staff. Clear, robust, flexible and responsive support structures, and open communication between service users and the agencies involved with them are necessary to manage individual and organizational risk and anxiety. However, while risks inevitably exist and require active management, they are balanced by the potential benefits of facilitating peer support.

At the heart of peer support is the concept of 'epistemic trust' [19]. This is defined as 'that particular trust in the value of social knowledge that a potential "teacher" may have to offer the learner'. It links to the neuroscientific finding

[20] that learning takes place preferentially in the context of a relationship in which the 'teacher' is felt to be a trusted source of information and knowledge; and this trust is enhanced when knowledge is communicated in a way that signals its personal relevance to the individual. The development of a peer relationship in which the newly released person feels understood by someone who has successfully travelled further along his or her own journey into the community offers the potential to enhance learning from experience, as compared with similar 'knowledge' conveyed by a professional, whose engagement may feel less personally addressed. In addition, the supervisory and authority nature of relationships with professionals—however benign in the professional's eyes—can easily activate many service users' underlying representations of parental and authority figures, thereby increasing arousal and reducing the capacity to think (or 'mentalize') [21]. The peer relationship may therefore have a particular role to play in increasing openness to learning and absorbing the steps towards a prosocial lifestyle.

The difficulties that lead to personality disordered offenders becoming 'service users' also present problems in relation to meaningful user involvement. Common problematic personality traits often make collaborative engagement difficult. Sensitivity to judgement, humiliation, and negativity mean that social encounters of any kind can trigger strong emotional reactions that the person may find hard to manage. When antisocial thinking takes over, working relationships can suddenly become hierarchical and hostile. The need to feel in control in relationships can impair a constructive, shared approach to problem solving. Lack of a sense of agency can lead to feelings of powerlessness and vulnerability in the face of perceived demands and expectations, leading to dropout and avoidance.

Why we chose our direction

The OPD pathway services we co-deliver span a range of prison as well as community services, so we started by deciding on some principles to underlie all our service user involvement initiatives. These provide consistency, while also allowing flexibility for the users and staff in each service to respond to local needs and opportunities.

We began with the overarching aims of the OPD pathway—reduced reoffending, improved well-being, and workforce development—and the factors that contribute to desistance from offending, namely developing a new nonoffender identity, having a social role, and building positive relationships and social connections. This led to the development of four key aims underpinning the user involvement strategy:

- To provide equal access to and opportunity for user-led and user-involving activities for pathways service users across London
- To assist the development of skills and interests that enhance personal agency, self-esteem, and prosocial roles and identities
- To improve care of self and the capacity to care for others
- To facilitate positive relationships and social engagement with peers and others.

How we've done it

Our involvement of service users has been gradual and to some extent organic, rather than being carefully planned, and we think this has worked well. This process has enabled our users and staff to contribute fairly equally to the identification and implementation of ideas and initiatives. However, we have tried to establish a basic framework to ensure that new developments are properly supported and responsive to feedback.

The underlying model of all pathways services is concerned with relationships and their facilitating power. In the early stages of developing services, our focus was primarily on relationships between professionals and service users as the medium of change, with service users being involved through being given information, collaborative engagement in their own formulation and risk management planning (especially in the prison services), consultation, and feedback. As time has gone on, the level of participation has increased with the emergence of more active roles.

We were mindful also that high-risk, high-harm offenders are a diverse group, with a wide range of strengths, needs, resources and capacities, and that opportunities for involvement needed to extend to everyone. We therefore suggested a stepped model, with three levels of participation:

- Level 1: Participation without an active development role (e.g. participating in feedback sessions, focus groups, shared social and recreational activities). Travel expenses are paid for these activities, to mitigate financial obstacles to participation
- Level 2: Participation with an active service development role (e.g. facilitating groups, carrying out service evaluation research, delivering training). Participants are paid at the current 'living wage' for these activities
- Level 3: Active involvement in projects with outside agencies, with support from our services (e.g. involvement in recruitment and presentations). In these activities, which relatively few individuals are able to engage with, the outside agency is expected to reimburse the service user.

Governance and risk management

Maintaining safety and managing risk is of course as important in user involvement as in any other OPD pathway service or activity. In all pathway services the criminal justice agency holds the risk, and this forms the basis of the procedural security and governance policy for the user involvement programme. All service users who are actively involved in pathway projects are referred or supported by a professional—usually either their offender manager or a psychological therapist. The offender manager is always involved in decisions about whether and how someone will participate, including in the case of self-referrals. The person's principal risk factors and risk situations, and any licence conditions, are shared amongst the team, and openly discussed with the service user to ensure that there is a shared understanding of risks and how they will be dealt with. Each project has its own safety and risk management protocol, which sets out communication, recording, and support procedures, and how concerns or an increase in risk will be dealt with. This always includes communication with the offender manager, who is involved whenever there is a difficulty or concern. Staff follow up and debrief service users who have been involved in delivering any sort of intervention, and there is a regular support structure for peer mentoring, which includes individual support, peer feedback, and reviews involving the offender manager. The monthly user forum includes a structured feedback session which encourages communication of any difficulties as well as achievements, and provides the opportunity to share and problem solve difficult situations.

Prisons

In each of the prison services, this process has been largely integrated into existing structures, for example:

- Keywork sessions focus on developing a 'formulation', which is an opportunity for prisoners to work collaboratively with staff on building a shared understanding or 'story' of how they have got where they are today, to understand their own risk, and make sense of professionals' concerns.

- This has led to the development of groups and workshops in which prisoners learn about the basis of risk assessments, for example the Historical Clinical Risk Management-20 (HCR-20), and how to take responsibility for their own risk management by understanding their supervision licence as a negotiated contract between themselves and their supervisor.

- Prisoners chair their own three-monthly review meetings.

- 'Buddying' programmes have been set up to encourage peer support, particularly for new prisoners coming into the service, and experienced users are involved in induction meetings alongside staff.

- Prisoners are supported to act as co-facilitators in psycho-educational and skills groups, and to co-develop groups that have particular meaning for them—for example a 'Surviving Prison' group.

- The social/recreational activities element of the Psychologically Informed Planned Environments (PIPE) (see Chapter 5 for a description of PIPEs) has enabled service users to bring and develop their own ideas for communal activity, working together with staff and learning how to take responsibility for planning, organizing activities, and getting along with each other.

- Community meetings are a forum for bringing suggestions and collectively agreeing how to prioritize and take them forward.

- Prisoners have the opportunity to take on roles and responsibilities, for example chairing community meetings, organizing activities, and acting as representatives in decision-making work groups, including the Enabling Environments programme (see Chapter 5).

- Prisoners may work in partnership with staff at formal meetings to present quarterly reports, and plan and run open days for staff and visitors from inside and beyond the prison.

These initiatives have all effectively taken place within the 'boundary' of the prison in which the pathways service sits. We have also tried to bridge that boundary by inviting in former service users, who are now living in the community, to support others following behind them on the journey, either as volunteers or as paid employees. This model is common in other areas of health, such as drug and alcohol treatment, but has proved quite difficult to implement in pathways services. Prisons vary in their willingness to have former offenders in their establishment and the process of obtaining permission has ranged from uncomplicated to impossible. People who are still incarcerated do not necessarily welcome advice from peers who have gone out before them and may not want to hear about the struggle of community living. And for those who come back, returning to an environment they have left behind can be potentially destabilizing.

In recent years, the term 'expert by experience' has become common as a shorthand for people who are active in a service user movement. Our various experiences over the last four years have made us cautious about this term and about whether viewing anyone as an 'expert' in facilitating change in others is helpful. For a service user who takes on formal paid employment as a service user consultant, the challenges are considerable. He/she needs to have a range of qualities: personal experience of criminal justice or health services in order to have both credibility and an understanding of what is needed; a high level of self-awareness; the ability to identify and discuss difficulties openly; and the ability to use leadership and management skills in organizationally challenging and complex settings. This is a very big ask for any individual, however robust.

The whole pathways project is based on the notion of partnership. Our experience suggests that the most helpful approach to working alongside service users is to combine professional attention to the boundaries of user involvement activities (including support and oversight structures, and the negotiation of risk management concerns across agencies) with grassroots identification and development of ideas and initiatives to take forward.

Community

In the community we began by establishing a service user forum (see Box 6.1) to oversee all user involvement initiatives and agree new ideas and projects. The forum is made up of representatives of all the main stakeholders in London Pathways Partnership (LPP) services—service users, clinicians, and probation staff—and meets monthly. It reviews the different projects and discusses and plans further progress. The forum occasionally invites external professionals who take an active role in service user involvement elsewhere or who represent other services in line with the forum's interests and priorities. A service user chairs this meeting.

Box 6.1 Service user forum: Mark

I remember going to the first forum and starting to put together the mentoring course. From a personal point of view, it is a mix of developing the skills for myself and the organization. It gave me a focus and I felt that I had something to contribute. It also helped me with structure and travelling—and just being around people, as I had found this cripplingly difficult. I wanted to contribute and be part of the community at large. I had been involved in therapy for thirty years and this was invaluable but was a constant one-sided conversation. It didn't help me be around 'normal' people. Service user involvement has not had the same hierarchies and I have felt like I have been valued and listened to—but also had the opportunity to ask questions and feel like that was OK. It gave me a voice. This process has been cathartic for me—as I was developing and reclaiming my identity.

As time has gone on, the need for more attention to be paid to transitions between services and settings has become clear. People who return to the community after a long period in prison face enormous challenges, and user involvement initiatives have had a particular contribution to make in this respect, as Dan's and Si's stories illustrate (Box 6.2).

Box 6.2 Service user involvement: Dan and Si

Dan

The thing I like about service user involvement projects the most is that it caters for everybody. It doesn't have to be standing in front of people—it could be to be involved in meetings or the social enterprise. I think for me this is almost more important. For a lot of guys, part of the challenge is to open yourself up to that world and believe you have a worth and a voice in this world. I have found one of the most difficult things is the relationship side of things. You are almost entering the professional world and I am respected and listened to, but I still don't feel I fit in the social element of it, which has been a challenge to deal with. On one hand, you are there as an equal, but only during the professional forum and I would never be invited with everyone to the pub afterwards. So that is about learning about who you are and developing what is necessary about this unique role. It is actually quite healthy as you are a conduit between the two worlds. The whole idea is to bring the two worlds closer together and restrictions will be part of that. Staff have been so committed to the process and what we do and I have not seen this outside this forum.

Si

Isolation almost justified committing crimes. Having people believe in you and feel you are cared about means you belong to something—and for those of us who have never belonged to anything positive, it is frightening to think of letting yourself or others down—or losing the life you've built up and can start to feel proud of. It is a two-sided thing—it instils in you a sense of belief. Everyone always says you can do it. There isn't a 'wrong'—it is just to be open about who you are and what you think. It is transparent and it develops your ability to take on different perspectives and to have 'real-life', non-therapy-type conversations. It is not about what is impossible—it is about how to make it possible.

Pathway activities have tended to fall into one of four areas:

- Facilitating peer support and mentoring across the prison–community boundary
- Providing training for staff to help them better understand the challenges faced by service users
- Service evaluation to ensure users' experience of services is properly captured and influences future developments
- Consulting to staff teams about service-related issues, such as how to develop service user involvement across different contexts.

Individual initiatives are discussed below.

Peer mentoring

With professional support, a group of service users developed a peer mentoring training package and have trained up a group of peer mentors. Mentors are matched with mentees by staff after careful consideration of their respective histories, interests, and personality difficulties, and with the involvement of their probation officers. Mentees are usually still in custody or a secure hospital at the time of referral, and whenever possible at least one meeting with the mentor, supported by a professional, takes place before their release to the community. After release, the focus of the mentoring relationship is on providing support for present-day practical challenges, such as accessing benefits, registering with health agencies, and finding out what community resources are available (see Box 6.3).

Mentoring takes place weekly for an hour, mentors are paid, and mentees receive travel expenses. A professional from the health team provides a weekly debrief/supervision to mentors and a monthly review with each mentor–mentee

---

Box 6.3 Peer mentor: Dan

I called my mentee recently and he said he had intended to call me the next day. We spoke for a good thirty minutes and he did most of the talking. Being there for someone is so satisfying, priceless. Often that is all that's required, a 'listening ear'. Not feeling alone or abandoned is vital. I call my mentee at least once a week and we meet once a week too, and he finds it very useful. To be able to do this is incredibly rewarding for me. My self-confidence has grown in leaps and bounds. I am a lot more stable now and less likely to reoffend or to become so depressed. Feeling that I am a part of someone's rehabilitation is just so satisfying.

pair, and liaises closely with offender managers throughout to ensure any risk issues are addressed promptly.

'Forward Thinking' group

Service users and staff designed the 'Forward Thinking' group which is now jointly delivered by a service user and a staff member in Approved Premises across London (see Box 6.4). The programme focuses on stress management during the period of transition from prison to the community, as well as practical issues such as housing and benefits.

Some service users who are 'treatment graduates' also provide regular peer support to participants in a national mentalization-based treatment (MBT) programme, helping to assess referred clients and sharing their own experience to relieve anxieties and assist with engagement.

Third-party disclosure training

Third party disclosure has become the norm rather than the exception for sexual and violent offenders subject to Multi-Agency Public Protection Arrangements (MAPPA). Disclosing a past violent or sexual offence to a potential employer, training organization, or new partner is a significant hurdle faced by offenders when they are trying to establish themselves in the community, and many end up leading restricted and impoverished lives either because of a negative outcome after disclosing or because they prefer not to take the risk. A group of service users and staff have been trained in all aspects of managing disclosure by a non-statutory criminal justice charity, and now deliver workshops tailored to this sub-group of offenders in pathway services, both custodial and community (see Box 6.5). The workshops not only focus on disseminating factual information but also seek to provide an opportunity to explore the complexities involved in disclosing to different people in different contexts.

Box 6.4 'Forward Thinking' group co-facilitator: Charlie

I found co-facilitating this group at an Approved Premises hostel very challenging at first, but then very rewarding. Not many people attended, but those who did found my input useful, especially as they could identify with me as I had 'been there, done it' so they could not pull the wool over my eyes! They always listened to what I had to say and I was able to support the member of staff I co-facilitated with when things became difficult. This was incredibly empowering and gave my self-confidence a real boost.

Box 6.5 Disclosure training co-facilitator: Henry

Delivering the disclosure training has been more of a challenge, but equally rewarding. As I am fond of saying, if we can reach just *one* person it has been worthwhile. We have done this a few times at different venues including hostels, a social inclusion project, and in a prison. My experience of running the workshop in the prison was a challenge (going back into prison for the first time as a visitor!). The member of staff I co-facilitated with made it very easy for me, and although the group was mixed and not the easiest, I left feeling that we had made an impact. Some of the inmates found what we had to say distressing, but I was able to remain calm and focused which helped. From my own experience I know that disclosure is a huge stumbling block, in particular for lifers, so I really wanted to 'succeed' in sharing the training I had on this topic.

Teaching and training

Service users join with professionals to deliver training both to pathways staff and to others in the wider health and criminal justice systems. Participants in these training events have so far included volunteers from third-sector agencies, students on professional training courses, prison officers, probation officers, social care staff, psychological therapists, and commissioners (see Boxes 6.6, 6.7 and 6.8). We have also supported service users to train with a third-sector organization and complete the 'train the trainers' course for the Personality Disorder–Knowledge and Understanding Framework (KUF) awareness training (see Chapter 2 for a more detailed explanation of KUF).

Box 6.6 Staff training: Reg

It was so nerve-wracking at first, but I went to speak to psychologists and probation officers about my life, my childhood, drinking, offending .... I then told them about what I am doing now. It felt quite overwhelming—I feel like I was doing a lecture and people actually wanted to listen to me and then thanked me. Words can't describe it. I want to give back to society, but people like me have been seen as less than animals. As nothing. Hated. When I spoke to this group, they said they were able to have a different view. I can't tell you how lovely it was to have someone with 'brains' come and say you helped them think differently.

Box 6.7 Training: Adam

We spoke to service users and a lot of probation staff, and having them hanging off every word was a real buzz for me! And to hear the feedback afterwards was just so rewarding and uplifting. I am very excited about the next one! Just to be able to get the message out there that there *is* hope and that men/women *can* succeed is really satisfying.

Service evaluation

Several service users have been trained to interview other users, enabling them to carry out both face-to-face and telephone interviews as part of service evaluations. The next step is for service users to conduct focus groups, engage in the process of thematic analysis, review results and recommendations, contribute to preparing evaluation reports, and present findings to commissioners or wider audiences.

Social enterprise

In a partner project—a high-support hostel for personality disordered offenders which is run as a partnership between health, probation, and social care staff—service users have developed a social enterprise project with its residents. This has developed a range of regular, small-scale projects, including regular catering, market stalls, provision of an 'Easy Read' service, and providing training to professionals (see Boxes 6.9 and 6.10). Any profit is ploughed back into the social enterprise for further development. The narrative in Box 6.9 portrays the experience of one of the residents at the hostel and the impact of the project on his life more widely.

Box 6.8 Training and lectures: Phil

During my talks to services and conferences, I was able to talk about my life and childhood in a way where 'I' wasn't a demon in the cupboard anymore. I needed to reclaim myself somehow rather than have my life in segments. SUI [Service user involvement] helped make me 'whole' and being a balance between the different parts of myself .... The external talks are so important to me because I hope it gives people an insight into how my life is much richer than the worst parts of myself. It also helps with relationships as it is about trust.

Box 6.9 Social enterprise at the hostel: Charlie

I was released from prison to the hostel, and at first I wondered how I would manage, amongst other things. I did not need to worry but didn't know that then! Once I grasped the ethos of the hostel, I knew it was the right place for me. I had so much support from the staff team, especially when I was extremely low in mood (having had a serious suicide attempt in 2013). If it wasn't for the hostel I would most likely have taken my own life. I loved the Thursday Programme, as it was then, especially the MBT group, and the one-to-one work with staff. Gradually I began to turn my life around, and metamorphosed into someone new, who had hope and a new-found confidence.

Once the saga of the PIP [disability benefit] was sorted out, I began to 'blossom' into the more mature and rounded man I am today. I joined in activities to help with the social enterprise, baking for the Xmas Market, and loved it. This has since blossomed into a proper 'enterprise' and we now bake goods for the Quakers and they sell our products in their café. Going to the hostel was the best thing that ever happened to me.

Café Project

In partnership with a third-sector organization, the Café Project was set up in 2013 in a central London café, offering a weekly supported space for isolated service users to socialize with one another, and learn and practise new skills such as cooking and art. The primary aims included a reduction in social isolation and an improvement in self-agency, confidence, and interpersonal functioning. The project is constantly evolving and now provides sessions on healthy eating, yoga, and creative writing, plus a variety of educational workshops,

Box 6.10 Social enterprise at the hostel: Glen

At the hostel I was working with the staff as a maintenance rep, and chaired several meetings between the clients and staff. I was in charge of the 'bank' for the social enterprise group and for a while worked with the staff on the client's budget regarding outings and birthdays, etc. All this gave me the skill to be a responsible person, not only for others but also for myself and my own life events, to make sure, as best as possible, that the hostel ran smoothly.

Box 6.11 Café Project: Reg

I have got a lot of enjoyment out of it—particularly because it has boosted my cooking skills and my confidence so much. It is a friendly atmosphere and I always get on with everyone—staff and service users. For most of my life I was put down and told that I was an idiot and I would never be anything and you believe that is who you are. [The Café Project] has been part of what has helped me think a bit differently about myself. It has given me a lot of confidence—through helping out first of all and feeling like I have people around me who are supporting me.

I now feel like I can motivate others, and it has gone full circle where I can help others as I have been helped. I feel like I belong to something that is meaningful and I guess that makes me feel that I have more to offer than I ever thought. That feels amazing. I am now the church warden and I feel like I am trusted because they got to know me through [the Café]. I feel appreciated and more confident about the future. I don't think I would ever offend again because I don't want to go back to how I was. I feel like I belong to something new and positive and don't want to lose that. I like my life and my friends, and being part of [the Café] has encouraged me to branch out into new groups, like the church, the choir, and another support group. I got to go with the church to Cambridge and I would never have done something like that if I didn't have the confidence I have now.

some hosted by service users on topics such as disclosure and welfare benefits. Two service users sit on the partnership steering group and service users take a lead on planning and reviewing activities (see Box 6.11). The narrative in Box 6.11 highlights the experience of one service user who, like many others, has used the Café Project as a platform from which to spring into a number of different prosocial roles.

Evaluation and learning

Each of our service user involvement initiatives is regularly reviewed as part of a reflective development process, with learning as far as possible being fed back into the project's development as it has continued forward. Service users write and present feedback on the projects, as well as contributing to steering groups, project committees, and the service user forum. In line with our contractual reporting cycle, they now produce a quarterly report identifying activity, achievements, and challenges. Some of the overarching lessons so far are discussed below.

Peer relationships and personal boundaries

Our experience, thus far, of observing and supporting the development of peer relationships has demonstrated the contribution of this support both to desistance from offending and to quality of life. Mentees report feeling less judged, more able to express themselves in their own words, and as experiencing a sense of optimism as they recognize change. Mentors say that the experience of feeling needed has helped them to perceive themselves as role models and as potentially useful citizens. This experience represents the most commonly reported motivation for deciding to be, and remain, a mentor.

Challenges have included mentors feeling helpless, perhaps carrying an inflated sense of responsibility for supporting the mentee's transition; mentors feeling overwhelmed by a 'déjà vu' sense of reliving the early stages of their own personal journeys; and the boundary around the mentoring relationship slipping as the two become more intertwined in a friendship. These experiences have highlighted the importance of regular supervision and reviews in which the progress of the relationship is transparently discussed, and it becomes the norm to work through difficulties rather than avoiding them or acting them out.

Managing stigma

Users of pathways services have themselves often been victims, and when they return to the community they continue to face the stigma of a serious offence history. Those who deliver training to professionals sometimes hear very negative comments about personality disordered offenders, which can feel extremely personal in an already demanding and stressful situation. Preparing service users for these experiences and debriefing and supporting them after any training event, as well as addressing any such incidents with the professional concerned, are essential. Messages from the professional network that appear to dismiss or cast doubt on the possibility of a former offender living as a law-abiding citizen have the potential to escalate risk and need to be managed sensitively at an organizational level. Similarly, service users have experienced threatening remarks from other service users (e.g. 'Who's side are you on?'). These interactions demonstrate the importance both of staff supporting service users in their new roles and of service users having their own robust coping mechanisms.

Who is the 'expert'?

There is a well-established model of employing a paid service-user consultant to support user involvement in health settings (including secure health settings). Where the shared service user experience is of personality disorder, individuals who put themselves forward for such a role, and who appear best suited to it, will not necessarily be (or be seen as) representative of others with the same diagnosis or clinical profile, particularly those whose primary 'public' identity is as an offender. A service-user consultant without a serious offending history may struggle with the antisocial presentation of offender peers and with the exposure to others' high level of trauma. Many people with personality disorder have themselves been victims of abuse, and exposure to perpetrators of physical and sexual violence (who also frequently have abuse histories) is potentially retraumatizing. User-led organizations for people who have been through the criminal justice system have to be sensitive to a variety of potential risks, and may be most accessible to those with less serious and/or less socially and politically sensitive offences. Our experience has shown that even a service-user consultant with experience of both personality disorder and offending may find the barriers to engagement in a prison setting just too difficult to manage.

Formulation sharing

Empowering users by developing a shared understanding of their psychological difficulties and risk remains central to the OPD pathway approach, and some attempts to do this—for example actively involving prisoners in understanding the HCR-20 and their own risk assessments—have been clearly successful, with high levels of engagement by prisoners and improved understanding and 'ownership' of their risk. However, the collaborative development of a 'formulation' of the offender's personality, which is a cornerstone of the pathways approach, has remained quite problematic. There are external standards for these formulations, which aim to ensure they meet the requirements for communication amongst professionals (particularly psychologists and probation officers—see Chapter 3 for more details), but the extent to which formulations are understood by, and are meaningful to, the offenders and other non-specialist staff is still unclear. A study to explore the understanding and perceived usefulness of formulations in prison settings is underway, but how best to involve users in developing more effective ways to understand, manage, and communicate their personality difficulties and risk remains work in progress.

Risk management

Working in partnership with probation staff has been central to supporting all our service users in their active roles. The service user's offender manager holds the risk throughout, and the support of health staff, while integral to effective risk management, is essentially about adding value. In the peer mentoring programme, the mentoring relationship is regularly reviewed with the offender managers of both mentor and mentee. Service users need the support and understanding of their offender managers to succeed in these roles; this involves recognizing both improvements and dilemmas and risks that naturally crop up along the way. For example, service users wanting to go for a drink together, or confiding in one another about their offending histories, or sharing their home addresses have all been important issues to discuss openly in three-way meetings involving the service user, their offender manager, and LPP staff.

Supporting the management of their interpersonal world

Service users can feel very enthusiastic about helping others and are keen to get involved immediately, but it can be difficult for some to put their enthusiasm into practice. Fluctuations in their moods and general emotional instability—sometimes triggered by external factors and life stresses, sometimes by internal factors—can derail their ability to get involved and sustain a regular commitment. This can lead to 'approach-avoidance' patterns, which users need the help of staff to reflect on and manage. We have learned that what, on the surface, looks like unreliability is often an inner tug-of-war between the 'old me' and 'new me'. Supporting service users to articulate this conflict helps them to develop their own agency and reliability.

Excluding those with sexual convictions

All our projects involve service users with histories of violent and/or sexual convictions, and we have observed the emergence of sub-groups based on offence type. A perceived 'hierarchy' of offending, with sexual offenders at the bottom of the pecking order, is commonplace in criminal cultures, and a small number of service users with violent convictions have said they will refuse to work alongside those they believe have sexual convictions. In practice, there is generally a degree of tolerance, provided sex offenders are not explicitly identified, and we give a consistent message that user involvement activities are there to support all service users who want to make something different of their lives. However, we do need to be constantly mindful of the need to manage these tensions and associated risks.

Staff barriers

Despite persistent invitations, there has been some hesitancy amongst staff to attend and take an active interest in the service user forum. This is partly due to workloads and the time needed to attend (half a day, when travel is taken into account), but feeling out of one's 'comfort zone', and being unsure how to relate to service users on a more equal footing, is also a factor. However, over time, a growing number of probation staff and psychological therapists have attended the forum and volunteered to introduce service-user involvement to their teams.

Power dynamics

Occasionally we have observed some staff and service users get drawn into polarized positions in which service users vent their frustrations with the criminal justice system and staff react defensively. For instance, many of our service users have had previous negative experiences of leaving prison and moving into hostel accommodation, and some feel very passionate about their experiences of neglect and poor treatment at this difficult time in their lives. The forum has witnessed several heated debates between service users and staff on the sorts of reforms that should take place in hostels. However, despite the discomfort of these debates, in which power differences are very evident, they have sparked off useful and proactive initiatives, such as the 'Forward Thinking' group, the development of 'Welcome' packs for new residents, a buddy system, and direct engagement with residents' meetings.

How representative are they?

The majority of service users who are involved in the projects we have described are particularly invested in self-change and improving the lives of others. Initially they were mainly white, middle-aged men who had spent lengthy periods in custody. This group tended to volunteer themselves for most of the work, whether group facilitation, peer mentoring, or service evaluation. Although they may not be representative of personality disordered offenders as a whole, they represent one end of the resettlement pathway, having already processed a significant amount of change and being ready to support it in others. However, as time has gone on, we have had increased involvement from younger and minority ethnic service users who have recently 'graduated' from pathway services and who bring particular insights into how to engage their peers.

We have also learned that it is a misperception to believe that just because someone has a diagnosis of a personality disorder, they represent others with a personality disorder or are well suited to supporting others with similar difficulties. Observing service users struggle to engage other service users, and even be ridiculed for it, has highlighted the need to think carefully about 'matching' people in mentoring relationships, and generally create an atmosphere that respects difference, is tolerant of interpersonal stress, and provides robust support structures in which difficulties can be shared openly.

Personal change

As a staff team we have been impressed by the impact of involvement initiatives on service users' internal world and resettlement journeys. We have seen them develop confidence and skills and meet daunting challenges with integrity and commitment. These changes are best expressed in the service users' own words (see Boxes 6.12, 6.13, and 6.14).

Next steps

Earlier in this chapter we commented that the gradually increasing involvement of service users has been largely organic, evolving as both staff and users have learned how to work effectively in partnership with each other. This process has been underpinned by principles rather than strategy. On the basis of our learning so far, there are now some clearer aims for the next phase.

Consolidation and strengthening of work done so far

An important strand of development will involve strengthening and deepening the work done so far, engaging actively with challenges and dilemmas, and ensuring that governance and support structures keep pace with increasingly demanding and complex activities. We plan to extend all the activities described in this chapter: training more peer mentors (there are more potential mentees than mentors at present); developing training and educational activities, both within the pathway and with workers from outside agencies; delivering workshops to other service users; embedding service users in treatment groups as facilitators and peer supporters; supporting increased ownership of the Café

Box 6.12 Personal change 1

... it's empowering and you feel important rather than just a bystander ... that you 'matter', which for many of us is a 'first', having been just a number for so long ... .

Box 6.13 Personal change 2

Feeling that I am a part of what happens to me and others is very important, as for most of my life I had no say in my fate and it was always behind closed doors.

Project by service users; and developing a more systematic programme of user-led evaluation of the pathway services we co-deliver.

Improving engagement of more hard-to-reach service users in all aspects of the services we co-deliver

Now that pathways services are well established, a primary aim is to make them accessible to all those who may benefit. We believe that service users have a key role to play in identifying the barriers to some individuals engaging in pathway services, such as those who are younger and from minority groups. To this end, we have started a consultation process with a group of minority ethnic service users to generate a plan for overcoming these barriers in both prisons and the community.

Box 6.14 Personal change 3

I am always aware that I have PD and this brings challenges. I feel being meaningfully involved in the world around me has given me a really good tool kit. With the right staff support you really start to contribute in the quality of your own life and the life of others. It stops you feeling so disconnected. I also feel I have a right to tell my story—despite all the negatives, I now believe there are things that are positive about me. This resonates for me as a person, as I have always focused on what I can't do—and prison has been like that.

It is important to feel you have choices—I feel like I am living my life now and the pathway is so important because it doesn't feel abstract. I have structure with clear initiatives and a role.

I felt like the people around me have supported me and this support structure reinforces the positive. It is much easier for me to accept criticism—I've always known that, but accepting praise has been a really important thing. It helps me to develop and see and value the best of myself.

Establishing effective user representation

Tokenism has bedevilled the user-involvement movement. We are therefore planning a scoping exercise involving both users and staff, to look at what has and hasn't worked well in other settings, and to identify a model of representation on management and decision-making groups that is effective, realistic, and sustainable. Our co-delivery of several different services provides the opportunity for applying a model consistently and establishing peer support mechanisms for those involved.

New developments

Following service users across the prison–community boundary has highlighted to us both the impact of imprisonment—in which people not infrequently suffer and witness traumatizing levels of aggression, violence, and manipulation—and the disorientation of release into the community. It can take weeks or months for any significant adjustment to occur, particularly after a long sentence and when the person has no support network to rely on. The LPP's third-sector partnerships (see Chapter 4) offer support with practical issues, and our peer mentoring scheme also aims to help with this transitional stress. Prompted by service users' own feedback—and their desire to try to mitigate some of the damage they see the prison environment causing—we are exploring the possibility of a more therapeutic intervention, involving service users, that could span the pathway from prison to the community and offer some preparation for the emotional consequences and demands of release.

Summary

It is all too easy to become disenchanted with the limitations imposed by traditional risk management models on an individual offender's opportunity to reintegrate into the community. The service-user voices in this chapter should give us grounds for optimism: personal cognitive transformation and increased social capital—the two core constructs of desistance theory—are clearly evident in their contributions.

Although we still think in terms of a 'London Pathways service-user involvement programme', the experience of developing it has highlighted to us that service users are also true partners in what we do and we are mutually engaged in a common project. Professionals who are committed to supporting user involvement in the OPD pathway often need to draw on the qualities that have been identified as necessary for working with personality disordered offenders generally, such as an ability to be compassionate and interested, to work collaboratively, being resilient in the face of mistakes and setbacks, and responding rather than reacting to difficulties. What is very striking to us is the capacity of the users themselves to draw on and develop similar qualities, and indeed at times to demonstrate a humbling level of tolerance, acceptance, and persistence in the face of enormous social and emotional stress. The fundamental rules of working with people with personality disorder apply in user involvement as much as any other activities: be transparent, apologize for mistakes, do what you say you'll do. Professionals frequently think about how to engage potential users in services; we also need to think about how to engage staff in user-led initiatives. We want users to listen to us; they want us to listen to them. Inevitably there are areas of challenge and of potential risk and conflict, but the same is true between partner agencies involved in the pathway, and they are manageable in the same way. Supported by effective communication and clear, robust governance and management structures, user involvement can be an integral part of working towards the overarching pathway aims of reducing reoffending, improving psychological well-being, and developing the workforce.

References

1. **Sainsbury Centre for Mental Health.** An evaluation of mental health service user involvement in the re-commissioning of day and vocational services. London: Sainsbury Centre for Mental Health; 2016.

2. **Department of Health.** Putting people first: planning together—peer support and self-directed support. London: Department of Health; 2016. http://www. thinklocalactpersonal.org.uk/_assets/resources/personalisation/personalisation_advice/ pt_final.pdf.

3. **Giddens A.** Modernity and self-identity: self and society in the late modern age. Cambridge: Polity Press; 1991.

4. **Department of Health.** A National Service Framework for mental health. London: Department of Health; 2016. https://www.gov.uk/government/uploads/system/ uploads/attachment_data/file/198051/National_Service_Framework_for_Mental_ Health.pdf.

5. **Wanless D.** Securing our future health: taking a long-term view. London: HM Treasury; 2016. http://www.yearofcare.co.uk/sites/default/files/images/Wanless.pdf.

6. **NHS England.** Transforming participation in health and care, guidance for commissioners. Redditch: NHS England; 2013. https://www.england.nhs.uk/2013/09/ trans-part/.

7. **Davies HTO, Nutley SM, Mannion R.** Organisational culture and quality of health care. Quality in Health Care. 2000;9(2):111–119.

8. **NHS England.** Improving experience of care through people who use services. Redditch: NHS England; 2015. https://www.england.nhs.uk/wp-content/uploads/2013/ 08/imp-exp-care.pdf.

9. **Arnstein SR.** A ladder of citizen participation. Journal of the American Institute of Planners. 1969;35(4):216–224.

10. **Byrne L, Happell B, Reid-Searl K.** Lived experience practitioners and the medical model: worlds colliding? Journal of Mental Health. 2016;**25**(3):217–223.

11. **Godin P, Davies J, Heyman B, Reynolds L, Simpson A, Floyd, M.** Opening communicative space: a Habermasian understanding of a user led participatory research project. Forensic Psychiatry and Psychology. 2007;**18**(4):452–469.

12. **Hodge S.** Competence, identity and intersubjectivity: applying Habermas's theory of communicative action to service user involvement in mental health policy making. Social Theory and Health. 2005;**3**:165–182.

13. **Maruna S.** Making good: how ex-convicts reform and rebuild their lives. Washington, DC: American Psychological Association; 2005.

14. **Bottoms A, Shapland J.** Reflections on social values, offending and desistance among young adult recidivists. Punishment and Society. 2011;**13**(3):256–282.

15. **McNeill F, Weaver B.** Giving up crime: directions for policy. Glasgow: Scottish Centre for Crime and Justice Research; 2007. http://www.sccjr.ac.uk/publications/giving-up-crime-directions-for-policy/.

16. **Nugent B, Schinkel M.** The pains of desistance. Criminology and Criminal Justice. 2016;**17**:1–17.

17. **Weaver B.** Control or change? Developing dialogues between desistance research and public protection practices. Probation Journal. 2014;1–19.

18. **McNeill F.** Punishment as rehabilitation. In G Bruinsma and D Weisburd (Eds.), Encyclopedia of criminology and criminal justice. New York: Springer Science and Business Media; 2014, pp. 4195–4206.

19. **Fonagy P, Allison E.** The role of mentalizing and epistemic trust in the therapeutic relationship. Psychotherapy. 2014;**51**(3):372–380.

20. **Gergely G.** The development of understanding self and agency. In U Goswami (Ed.), Blackwell handbook of childhood cognitive development. Oxford: Blackwell; 2004, pp. 26–46.

21. **Bateman A, Fonagy P.** Mentalization based treatment for personality disorders: a practical guide. Oxford: Oxford University Press; 2006.

Chapter 7

The Offender Personality Disorder pathway: Modelling collaborative commissioning in the NHS and criminal justice system

Mick Burns, Colin Campbell, and Jackie Craissati

Introduction

One of the key underpinning principles of the Offender Personality Disorder (OPD) pathway is that of shared ownership, joint responsibility, and joint operations. This means that responsibility for individuals who meet criteria for the pathway is shared between the National Health Service (NHS) and Her Majesty's Prison and Probation Service (HMPPS), and services are jointly delivered within a collaborative culture in which partner organizations' respective knowledge, skills, and experience are valued [1]. Within the OPD pathway, this principle applies not only to the development and delivery of services but also to the commissioning of services.

There are numerous potential obstacles to ensuring that this principle underpins service commissioning, development, and delivery in practice. The aims and core tasks of the two partner organizations clearly differ, with, arguably, an asymmetry in how they prioritize two key aims of the OPD pathway, namely a reduction in serious offending and improved psychological well-being. The capacity to understand, much less value, partner organizations' knowledge, skills, and experience is undermined by increasing demands on diminishing resources in both partner organizations as a result of reduced public service funding. In addition, significant and frequent organizational change can limit the resources that can be made available for developing collaborative ways of working with other organizations, which can be further limited by the need for partner organizations to rapidly familiarize themselves with the implications of such changes on partnership working.

The first part of this chapter explores how a single collaborative commissioning approach (which involves NHS and criminal justice commissioners jointly commissioning and co-financing services), underpinning the OPD pathway, attempts to model the positive, collaborative, relational approach expected of partner providers in health and justice settings and between staff and service users. In the second part, the authors comment on their experience of joint working in both prison and probation settings. While these comments and views are those of the authors, necessarily, they draw heavily on conversations with numerous criminal justice colleagues in the context of commissioning, developing, and delivering services since the implementation of the OPD strategy in 2011.

Commissioning OPD services

Introduction

Commissioning a pathway of services is a complex process. A highly specialized approach is required for complex individuals who present a high risk of sexual and/or violent harm to others and who are likely to have a personality disorder. This is further complicated by the need to deliver across a range of organizations and in both community and secure settings.

Since the late 1990s and the conception of the Dangerous and Severe Personality Disorder (DSPD) programme, much has been learned about effective practice with this population. Perhaps the most important element in all this endeavour has been the understanding that a systemic approach, involving partners from a range of providers, working to deliver a pathway of services in a range of settings, is more important than any single intervention [2, 3].

'Co-commissioners' for the OPD pathway are required to occupy a difficult boundary position between and within systems (e.g. the purchaser/provider system, health and criminal justice systems, and provider and regulatory systems), between organizations, and even between staff and the service users under their care/supervision. This complex dynamic means that commissioners have a challenging role to manage, acting both within and outside the various systems and often acting as a repository for the anxieties in the various systems [4, 5]. It is therefore important for commissioners to be aware of the potential for these tensions to interfere with delivery of the primary task and to attend to them through the careful management of relationships in the system. These systemic tensions highlight how important it is for co-commissioners to lead and manage the system in a collaborative, psychologically informed manner.

Background to the programme

In October 2011, the then UK Coalition government published its response to the public consultation on the OPD pathway. This resulted in the reallocation of resources from the DSPD programme to an innovative approach with new services along a pathway across community and secure care (prisons and hospitals). This new pathway and the services within it would be, primarily, jointly delivered by agencies in the criminal justice system and providers of mental health services. The pathway is now well established (although it is still regarded as developmental as there remains much to learn); however, the approach to the commissioning of these services is less well recognized.

In 2011 the DSPD programme was managed under the auspices of the Department of Health and the National Offender Management Service (NOMS), an agency of the Ministry of Justice, and reported jointly to directors and ministers for both departments (see Chapter 1). As well as oversight of the DSPD programme, the team developed policy and strategy for offenders with personality disorder. The adoption of a new and what seemed at the time to be a radical approach was probably successful as a result of a number of factors.

From the outset the strategy was strongly supported by directors in NOMS and the Department of Health. This was given extra momentum by the Bradley Report recommendation [6] that an evaluation of the programme should be undertaken and a new strategic approach developed for all aspects of personality disorder in the criminal justice system. While there were some doubts about the deliverability of the new programme, government ministers were willing to take the risk because the benefits were potentially so significant. The high-level outcomes were explicit, easy to understand, aligned to the overarching key objectives of the departments, and, of key importance, did not require any legislative change. This was also a time of increasing austerity and the prospect of delivering more without additional resource was highly attractive.

The public consultation was a condition before approval to implement was given. Perhaps not surprisingly, given the highly specialized area in which the consultation took place, there were fewer than 100 responses. However, almost every one of these was supportive. This was due to several factors. First, there was extensive discussion with service providers, academics, and other experts in the field before the consultation document was written. Key individuals were identified, partly to seek their views and partly to persuade and influence their thinking. Every opportunity was taken to speak at a conference or attend a loosely connected meeting. As a result, there was a broad understanding of what would be supported and where the key challenges would lie. Formal discussions were also held with prisoners and patients then residing in the DSPD services, which helped develop a service-user perspective of their needs, concerns, and wishes. Second, the focus of discussions was limited to *what* we wanted the new approach to look like and avoided *how* it might be delivered. This is an important distinction because in areas of significant organizational complexity and change, how something might be done can seem so difficult that it becomes impossible to think about it as something that can happen. Third, discussions focused on the principles that might underpin the strategic approach. At this stage of strategic development we were interested in a shared and common set of values that would underpin all the new services, irrespective of whether they were primarily in health or the criminal justice system. This focus also helped those people in services that would be affected by the change in the way money was used to think about the overall picture and not just their impact.

In October 2011, with the government's response to the public consultation published, the direction of the team developed from one with primary responsibility for policy and strategy into one with a principal task of commissioning.

A brief recent history of commissioning in the NHS and the criminal justice system

In 1991, following the 1989 White Paper 'Working for patients' [7], the UK Conservative government introduced legislation to promote competition between healthcare providers. This was achieved by separating NHS organizations into 'purchaser/provider' roles. District Health Authorities, established in 1982 to run local hospitals on behalf of the Department of Health, became purchasers of care and were mandated to buy health services from local hospitals on behalf of their local communities. The intention was for the new internal market to drive down price and improve the quality of services through economic market mechanisms.

In opposition, the Labour Party campaigned against marketization of the NHS, arguing that the 'internal market' had caused fragmentation. However, on gaining power in 1997, the 'New Labour' administration published an equally radical manifesto of reforms that rejected the old 'command and control' and 'internal market' models [8] and, in 2002 [9], laid the ground for the introduction of further market reforms. By 2002 the 'purchasers' of 1991 had evolved into 'commissioners'—commissioners who would help patients navigate a complex web of choice about which provider (including private providers) to use for a range of elective procedures. The new system was given additional leverage by the withdrawal of block contracts (which saw hospitals given annual blocks of money with little incentive to change practice) which were then replaced by a complex 'payment by results' system which rewarded providers for seeing and treating more patients, thus driving down waiting times in the process.

NOMS was created in 2004 following a review by Lord Carter [10]. Carter proposed three radical changes: first, that there should be 'end to end' management of each offender from first contact with correctional services to full completion of the sentence; second, that there should be a clear division between the commissioners of services and their providers; and third, that there should be 'contestability' amongst those providers, thus, he argued, increasing efficiency. At the heart of commissioning in both conventions is an annual cycle of planning and agreeing requirements of services that are set out in contracts or Service Level Agreements. While based on need, these have also reflected changes in national policy and political objectives: for example, introducing payment by results and the need to restructure as a result of a more difficult financial climate. While remaining committed to delivering a commissioning model, NOMS struggled with the divide between purchaser and provider, often finding itself responsible for both. For example, NOMS employed the custodial commissioners for public sector prisons and is the provider for public sector prisons.

This conflict was addressed through the creation of HMPPS on 1 April 2017. While the primary purpose of protecting the public remains, this new agency's responsibility is primarily for operational delivery, including a new Youth Custody Service. Commissioning responsibility has been transferred to the Ministry of Justice, with the department also responsible for policy development, standards, and scrutinizing performance. The OPD programme, despite its commissioning role, is located in HMPPS. This is partly due to the nature of the relationship between co-commissioners and operational service delivery in prisons and the National Probation Service (NPS).

The Health and Social Care Act [11] introduced by the UK Coalition government laid the ground to open up the NHS to competition from 'any willing' (qualified) provider. The much-feared explosion in private competition did not materialize, and against a backdrop of public concern in NHS hospitals prompted by a highly publicized systemic failure of care in an NHS general hospital trust (2013), and a change in Health Secretary, much of the focus in the NHS during the latter part of the coalition term and the subsequent Conservative majority governments has been on strengthening the role of the regulator (The Care Quality Commission) in the NHS [12] and encouraging providers to work collaboratively in networks on behalf of communities, rather than competitively [13].

The discipline of commissioning has struggled to establish itself as being credible in the NHS since its introduction as 'purchasing' in 1991 [14, 15]. Various theories have been put forward to explain this failure to thrive: lack of clarity around what commissioning is and does [15]; the NHS tendency to re-organize itself at frequent intervals, denying the discipline the chance to mature [14]; and lack of evidence about what skills and competencies commissioners require [16].

Despite this, the high-level policy framework, driven by changing demographics, has inexorably moved the healthcare system towards a model that reinforces the need for the health economy to be underpinned by robust commissioning [17]. The phenomena of 'triple ageing' (the older population has trebled in the last fifty years and will treble again in the coming fifty years) across the European Union [18], increase in expectation from users of healthcare services, and technological advances in medicine and medical devices mean that there is significant potential for the costs of health and social care to spiral out of control [17]. A strong commissioning framework is seen as vital in moving the English health system away from a reactive, provider-driven system towards a more proactive, preventative approach built around strong commissioning [15, 19].

What is commissioning?

Commissioning in publicly funded services is a simple cyclical process. Commissioners are responsible for assessing the needs of individuals or a population, planning services to meet those needs, procuring or contracting those services to meet the need, and then evaluating how well this has been done. The cycle then starts again (see Fig. 7.1).

The commissioning process begins by engaging with individuals, communities, and systems to understand what outcomes need addressing, while concurrently brokering partnerships to meet those needs. On the OPD pathway this means working closely with operational and clinical colleagues and service users to develop a detailed knowledge of what is needed and how services can be developed or harnessed to meet identified need. The more effectively this is organized the better the outcomes for the population.

Commissioners therefore use a combination of methods: public health and criminological approaches, drawing on epidemiological studies, population-based research, and local system information. Most importantly, commissioners need to engage with frontline operational staff, clinicians, and service users to understand how care operates within a given service, and how it might be improved. Drawing together operational and clinical staff from a whole pathway is an effective means of understanding how the system can be directed to achieve the best outcomes.

Whatever method is used to assess and understand need it is important to build relationships with staff and service users in order for them to engage in any planned changes. This requires leadership. Commissioners need to provide

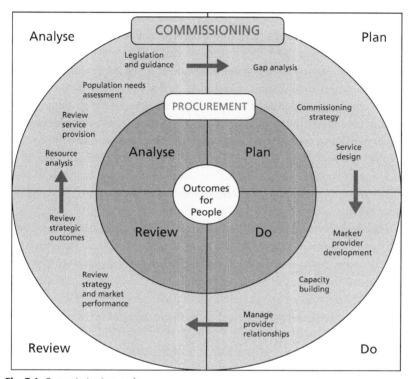

Fig. 7.1 Commissioning cycle

leadership within the system they are working with; sometimes this is a local system, sometimes a regional system, and on occasions it is across a national system. In whatever setting commissioning takes place the relationship with clinicians and service users will be instrumental in effecting change and this requires operational and clinical credibility, trust, and a vision of how things could change. The commissioner/provider relationship is complex; it is collaborative, not hierarchical, and dependent on a number of mutually agreed outcomes, some of which may require significant negotiation. The relationship is further complicated because it is usually transactional, in that it is driven through a contractual agreement, underpinned by a legal framework. In essence, however, the relationship is transformational and requires the commissioner to be able to develop and communicate a strategic vision for a pathway of services that providers want to subscribe to.

Establishing clear leadership allows commissioners to work in a collaborative way with clinicians, prison and probation staff, service users in provider organizations, and with other commissioners. In practical terms this requires commissioners to synthesize the views of clinicians, operational staff, other commissioners, and service users into a single vision and to develop a framework that can support the delivery of this vision in a consensual way.

Once we understand the outcomes that need to be addressed, a range of services then need to be planned and procured. This can involve the reorganization or refocusing of an established network of services, or it may require commissioners to innovate and to tender for new services. Commissioners need to be able to manage complex processes and projects to ensure that contracts are awarded in a way that avoids legal challenge while ensuring that service provision meets strategic objectives. It is not unusual for commissioners to plan in five- or even ten-year cycles in order to have the time to understand and re-design services to meet current and future needs.

Once providers have been contracted to provide a service, the contract then needs to be monitored. This process again requires significant collaboration with clinicians, managers, service users, and other commissioners to establish mechanisms by which the quality of services and the experience of those receiving the services can be measured. Commissioners are essentially responsible for managing this approach and holding providers of services to account on behalf of the public.

There is no universally recognized model of good practice for commissioning, in either health or criminal justice settings. The commissioning cycle as described above is well recognized, but attempts to standardize an approach to commissioning, such as the 'world class commissioning framework' (Box 7.1) [20] have failed to gain traction.

The commissioning approach described in this chapter is largely consistent with the model described above but differs in some subtle but very important aspects. Most commissioners are responsible for discrete areas of service provision, either an element of a pathway or a discrete geography. Commissioners on the OPD pathway are responsible for an entire pathway, which straddles custodial and in-patient services, and a range of community settings, both residential and non-residential. The commissioning framework is directly linked to high-level national strategy and the co-commissioners cover a much wider physical geography than commissioners would normally be expected to cover. The nature of the programme (something innovative that brings new money), the nature of the clinicians and practitioners working on the pathway (clinicians and practitioners who want to innovate and do things differently), and the fact that the pathway is co-commissioned from providers from different agencies working in partnership clearly brings a different dynamic to the commissioning relationship. The nature of the client group (high risk of harm and complex personality presentation), the complex nature of the organizations

---

Box 7.1 World class commissioning framework

World class commissioning will deliver

... better health and well-being for all—People live healthier and longer lives—Health inequalities are dramatically reduced.

better care for all—Services will be evidence-based and of the best quality, encompassing safety, effectiveness, and patient experience. People will have choice and control over the services that they use, so they become more personalized.

better value for all—Investment decisions will be made in an informed and considered way, ensuring that improvements are delivered within available resources—PCTs [primary care trusts] will work with others to optimize efficient and effective care.

---

within which the services are commissioned (prisons, the NPS, and the secure mental health system), and the previous difficulties encountered in commissioning appropriate services for this client group mean that a flexible transformative approach to service commissioning and service delivery is required. The key to this transformative approach is the notion of co-commissioning between NHS and criminal justice commissioners.

Co-commissioning

The OPD programme jointly commissions and co-finances its services; this is referred to as co-commissioning but, in reality, it is slightly more complex than the simple alignment of organizational objectives that this term normally refers to. Each of the four NHS England regions plus Wales has two commissioners, one from the NHS and one from HMPPS, working together to jointly commission a portfolio of services.

The primary focus is on the achievement of the programme outcomes, which, at their highest level, are expressed as public protection, psychological health improvement, workforce development, and the effective use of resources. The programme's principles underpin the strategic approach and therefore the commissioning approach. They provide, for commissioners and services, a shared philosophy—a way of thinking about the services that are delivered, how they are designed, and their operating models. The principles also provide a framework for decision making. They form a useful reference point against which difficult decisions can be made, including resource allocation, and tricky problems resolved. Using the principles helps prioritize competing options. Also provided are a set of common standards applicable to all services of the OPD pathway irrespective of type, model, security, or location.

The pathway consists of a range of service types, each described in a national, service-specific specification. The components of the pathway are rooted in the government response to the OPD consultation [21] as described below:

◆ The personality disordered offender population is a shared responsibility of HMPPS and the NHS.

◆ Planning and delivery is based on a whole systems approach across the criminal justice system and the NHS, recognizing the various stages of an offender's journey, from conviction, sentence, community-based supervision, and resettlement.

◆ Offenders who may attract the label 'personality disorder' who present a high risk of serious harm to others are primarily managed through the criminal justice system, with the lead role held by offender managers.

◆ Their treatment and management is psychologically informed and led by psychologically trained staff; it focuses on relationships and the social context in which people live.

◆ Related Department of Education and Department of Health programmes for young people and families will continue to be joined up with the OPD pathway to contribute to prevention and breaking the cycle of intergenerational crime.

◆ In developing services, account is taken of the experiences and perceptions of offenders and staff at the different stages of the pathway.

◆ The pathway will be evaluated focusing on risk of serious reoffending, health improvement, and economic benefit.

Services commissioned through the NOMS Commissioning and Commercial Directorate (from 1 April 2017, the Rehabilitation and Assurance Directorate in HMPPS) and NHS specialized commissioners have subsequently focused on:

◆ Improved targeting of resources for screening and early identification

◆ A focus on assessment, case formulation, and sentence planning

◆ Improving access to the high-security prison personality disorder treatment services

- Ensuring access to secure psychiatric hospitals for offenders with comorbid mental health problems where the requirements of the Mental Health Act are met and the NHS pathway is the most appropriate for the individual
- Developing personality disorder treatment units in category B and C prisons for men and closed prisons for women
- Improving access to existing accredited offending behaviour programmes, including democratic therapeutic communities in prisons
- Developing Psychologically Informed Planned Environments (PIPEs) in prisons and approved premises, which will provide offenders with progression support following a period of treatment or period in custody
- Increasing support for offender managers working in the community using established Multi-Agency Public Protection Arrangements (MAPPA) procedures.

There is an expectation that service design and delivery on the pathway is informed by evidence. However, services are encouraged to innovate, evaluate, and share learning, as over-reliance on established evidence can frustrate an innovative service response. What is important is to know what is known and the limitations and gaps in the evidence base. Many of the new services have been given three months to design their service. The service plans are considered and approved by commissioners before delivery commences.

The OPD programme's model of co-commissioning has common features applied nationally. Bringing together commissioners from different agencies brings with it differing organizational objectives but a shared responsibility for their achievement and a broader range of knowledge, skills, and experience. This enables co-commissioning from a team perspective, providing mutual support, one leading while the other observes, sense checking, and the opportunity to model expectations of the providers. The modelling of the key principles of shared responsibility and joint operations provides a reference point for provider partners on the pathway and facilitates building a psychologically informed relationship with providers, creating a sense of sharing ownership for the objectives and sharing responsibility for their effective delivery—'we are all in it together'. Throughout, we are trying to reach a common understanding of the challenges and how these might best be met. Historically, this population was managed either in the community, or in prison, or in hospital and responsibility was batted from agency to agency. Here, the intention is to work together as one organization, sharing the responsibility, difficulties, and successes. This should help to develop a shared understanding of problems and approaches to solving them. When problems occur, co-commissioners have a role in facilitating resolution; however, the differing authority that comes with one's own agency can be used to help reach such a resolution.

Underpinning the relationship with, usually, the senior managers of a service, prison governors, and assistant directors in the NPS is a relationship with service users and the staff who are operationally responsible from one day to the next. Contract meetings are usually preceded by discussions with service users about their experiences, the extent to which they understand why they are there and what they can reasonably expect, and whether key elements of the service are actually being delivered to them. Operational staff provide an informed view of what it is like to work in the service, the support and training they receive, and, a key test, the extent to which they understand the service model and their role within it.

As co-commissioners we have a responsibility for keeping an eye on the national picture. We provide a helicopter view of the system and the pathway that runs through it. The relationship between regional co-commissioners, with national thematic leads (for women, environments, and PIPEs) and with national professional networks, provides some consistency across regions to ensure that services develop equitably.

The importance of workforce and environments

The programme outcomes include the requirement to develop a capable and compassionate workforce (recognizing the significant demands associated with working with this difficult-to-reach population). This ambition was underpinned by a structured training framework (the Knowledge and Understanding Framework (KUF)) which was developed under the auspices of the Department of Health and Ministry of Justice through a partnership between Nottingham University, the Open University, Tavistock and Portman NHS Foundation Trust, and a Service User Organization 'Borderline UK' (latterly known as Emergence, but which went into liquidation in 2016). At the time, this provided the first national programme intended to raise awareness of personality disorder across health, criminal justice, and the third sector. This three-day training has been completed by more than 10,000 people. Additionally, more specialist and focused MSc and BSc modules became available.

As the OPD programme services have developed, more bespoke training has become available. Each provider partnership is expected to provide local training for staff tailored to the individual service area, for example, in the community, PIPEs, and treatment services. All this is supported by a robust supervision framework which is monitored through the contract framework, along with sickness/absence in services (sickness/absence is perhaps unsurprisingly low compared with national averages in public sector services and is, we think, reflective of the significant investment in the workforce). A practitioner guide [22] jointly produced by clinicians, operational staff, and co-commissioners has been developed and provides a key reference point for staff working along the pathway.

This investment has created a highly dynamic workforce across a range of services. There is in development a core model on which to base and conceptualize how the service delivers outcomes. This core model helps describe the known factors that can lead to offending and the complex psychological and social problems that can attract the label 'personality disorder'. There is, however, deliberately no overarching operating model for service delivery, and individual partnerships are required to develop clearly described approaches in response to the specifications. In addition, service delivery across the pathway is underpinned by a range of psychological models and approaches. The common denominator in all these approaches is the requirement to base plans (treatment plans, management plans, sentence plans) on a psychological formulation. The formulation provides a core around which different staff disciplines and the service users reach a shared understanding of what all parties are trying to achieve through the service delivery, and more importantly how this might be achieved. There is a high-level model for formulation with a range of levels (1–3, increasing in complexity) along with a set of standards and an audit tool for measuring the quality of the approach (see Chapter 3). The formulations are used to drive management plans, treatment, and interventions in some of the 'treatment' services, and to provide 'psychologically informed case management' across the rest of the pathway.

The whole programme is therefore based upon key pillars of a psychologically informed, well-supervised workforce, provision of enabling environments [23] (see Chapter 5) which will allow strong, healthy, therapeutic relationships to develop, and a consistent desire to see service users and staff feeding into the continual evolution of the individual service and the wider pathway.

Service partnerships are encouraged to innovate (sometimes incentivized by extra investment) and to continually evaluate the impact of the programme on individuals, teams, and environments. This flexibility and creativity is seen as being essential to the whole endeavour and has generally been embraced by workforce and service users alike. The joint approach to commissioning and service delivery is the most important element in realization of the programme objectives. The synthesis of clinical and operational expertise and the pooling of experience provide a rich platform from which to deliver an innovative service. However, partnership working is difficult. It is not sufficient for clinical and operational staff to work closely together on the frontline; it is equally important for organizations to align their strategic objectives to ensure that competing organizational priorities do not interfere with effective service delivery. Organizational tension frequently intrudes on the commissioning relationship and requires continual attention. In a small number of situations where an individual organizational priority has taken precedence, the service has failed. Co-commissioners and partner organizations have to continually negotiate this dynamic to ensure coherence of service delivery.

Evaluation

Achieving effective use of resources is one of the four key outcomes the programme has been tasked with achieving. A number of independent national evaluations have been commissioned. This is naturally a complex endeavour; evaluating the impact of a range of disparate psychological approaches on over 20,000 complex individuals across over 100 service settings delivered by over 2,000 staff could not be anything else. Individual partnerships are encouraged to evaluate their elements of the programme at a local level to inform the whole. As with all other elements of the pathway, this has required a flexible and innovative rather than a cautious and conservative approach. It is of paramount importance that as service models develop and evolve, as the workforce develops in its confidence and sophistication, and as service users progress along a pathway, the evaluation is sensitive enough to capture this.

This complex and dynamic network of service provision, underpinned as it is by an evolving psychologically informed workforce working with a group of extremely complex individuals, requires an equally complex and dynamic level of system leadership—leadership that is collaborative, flexible, and transformational in nature. The co-commissioning relationship that bridges the NHS and HMPPS approach to managing and treating complexity when it presents through the prism of 'high-risk personality disorder' provides the systemic environment in which this work can evolve.

The experience in prison

One of the key relationships in the development of OPD services in prison settings is that between 'new', largely NHS employed staff working in the OPD service and established prison staff, which include HMPPS psychologists and mental health in-reach staff. Arguably, this is particularly important in the development phase of the service when an understanding of each partner's experience and ways of working is developed; key working relationships are formed; and when it is crucial that a sense of joint ownership of the service, including both its delivery and outcomes, is developed. A joined-up approach to service design is essential to achieve a functional model of service delivery, while ensuring that the best use is made of the full range of experience and expertise in the design team.

An example of where this relationship was particularly important was in the development of an OPD service based on an outreach model in a Young Offender's Institution (YOI). In jointly developing this service, the objective of integrated working had to take account of the points of view of, and local contractual arrangements with, various stakeholders and partners. Without holding those relationships in mind, the development of the staffing and service model would have been stymied by potentially overlapping, unhelpful, and unnecessary aspects to the service (see Box 7.2 for a summary of findings). Knowledge and understanding of all those relationships helped to avoid conflict and dispute locally and any distraction from the clinical task. Stakeholders included the prisoners, the governing governor and his senior management team, the operational staff group, the primary and mental health care staff group, the HMPPS psychology staff group, and the commissioners themselves.

The approach to the design of the new service was very much based on the 'principles' and 'standards' of the OPD pathway (see Chapter 1). With an emphasis on joint design and collaboration, it seemed likely that the needs of multiple stakeholders and perspectives could be met, and ultimately the work needed to achieve this was one of the most significant tasks in getting the prison ready for the new service.

Stokoe's [24] suggested principles for healthy organization and teamwork held true in the design of the new OPD service (see Box 7.3). From the start, it was important for the design team to agree what the primary task of the service was going to be; to agree the various roles and responsibilities in the team; to provide clarity about the operational principles of the work; and to consider how to ensure thinking space was provided to the team in a context that supported reflective practice. The members of the design team had sufficient experience and expertise in service design in providing services to young adult males and in custodial settings to be alert to the problems that can occur when the task is not clear: for example, security versus therapy in a secure unit setting, or when managers are not given enough authority to carry out their role, or when the issue of boundary management is not attended to—true surely in any caregiving team but especially so when working with those given a personality disorder diagnosis [25].

As described earlier in the 'Background to the programme' section, the focus of the service development discussions was about *what* the prison and team wanted the new approach to look like and not *how* it was going to be delivered at any early point. When developing a service for emerging personality disorder in young adult men in custody, it was a large advantage to be able to develop a

Box 7.2 Outline of the YOI OPD pathway needs analysis and model design

- The YOI in which the OPD service is located is responsible for holding a particularly challenging and high-risk young adult [18–21 year-old] population. It holds the longest-sentenced young male offenders in the prison system, including a large number of young adults serving life and indeterminate sentences. 'The behaviour of some of these young adults is very challenging, others are very vulnerable, and plenty are both' ([37], p. 5).

- In preparation for the OPD service being commissioned, a needs analysis of the population identified that 32% of the population met the Offender Assessment System (OASys) criteria for possible personality disorder (see Chapter 3 for further details), 37% were identified as high risk on static risk measures for future violent and general offending, and 17% met both the personality disorder and high-risk criteria [37].

- The new OPD service therefore had to be able to respond to a population with high levels of trauma and neglect, disrupted attachments in relationships, loss and bereavement issues, intellectual difficulties, and neurological problems as a result of acquired brain injury, as well as the usual challenges in adolescence of the necessary cognitive, emotional, and relational developments.

- The following basic principles were adopted for service design:
  - Full integration and collaboration with the entire prison
  - A simple model of care understood by staff and young men
  - Training and space for staff reflection across the establishment to up-skill the whole workforce in managing difficult prisoners
  - An evolving treatment service, focusing initially on in-reach work with identified young people, building towards offering intervention and a more comprehensive therapy programme later on
  - To link with pre-existing services in the YOI to work towards those in treatment progressing through their sentence plan and accessing resources available locally.

> ## Box 7.3 Stokoe's four factors for a healthy organization
>
> 1. Clarity about the primary task (what we are all here to do)
> 2. Clarity about shared principles (how we set about the primary task)
> 3. Clarity about the different layers in the hierarchy, specifically what decision making is delegated to each level and with what authority
> 4. The factor that is specific to our work is the provision of a 'container'; this requires attention to something that does not arise in business—the management of 'good practice'.

bespoke service for this particular YOI, as there is a lack of theory and evidence available to guide such specific discussions. It let the service development team draw on what was felt clinically useful and what would most likely work in the YOI.

Learning was taken from the early publications coming out of the then new, community-based services for personality disorder. For example, Price et al. [26] analysed the service structure and treatment process involved in the eleven pilot services set up to focus exclusively on the needs of people with personality disorder (non-forensic). The eleven services provided a broad range of different services to users, including general support and advice, psycho-education, and specific social, occupational, psychological, and medical interventions. The key themes arising from the evaluation were the need to combine psychological treatments with social interventions and opportunities for peer support, for clear boundaries that are shared by service users, and for service users to be involved in managing their crises and planning future service developments. The personal qualities of staff were felt by service users to be as important as qualifications: for example, to be emotionally mature, to have a positive attitude, to be able to discuss their own mistakes, and to work as part of a team. All of these findings map well onto Stokoe's key principles of healthy team functioning.

The strengths of the service design are that it aims explicitly to balance the need to address both the victim and perpetrator experiences of the young men in the YOI. Without a team of staff who are able to hold onto the '*both/and*' position referred to by Bion [27], the young man is not contained and usually seeks to act out the experiences and unresolved issues not being attended to. For example, a young adult with a forensic history of multiple acts of serious violence does not necessarily benefit if clinical effort is devoted only to helping him understand his own experiences as a victim of violence. The service has to hold in mind the constant need for balance of the prison's security perspective and the need for creative, therapeutic treatment, and ensure the whole staff team take responsibility for both clinical and operational tasks to model safe containment to the service user. So the mix of various health staff from psychology, occupational therapy, art therapy, and systemic therapy alongside officer- and manager-grade operational staff offered a variety and depth of skill mix, with a multitude of approaches, methods, and tools to be used depending on the need of the clients. From the start, good use was made of the University of College London competences [28] to guide the spread of knowledge and skills required in the team, and this continued to be useful as a helpful reference point in supervision of staff as the service developed.

The commissioners played a leadership role akin to Obholzer's [29] idea that the leader should enable his or her organization to manage change by being open to the outside world yet not overwhelmed by it, and by managing the 'osmotic' boundaries to allow for change and growth (akin to Stokoe's idea of a constant flow in how the team works, where information is absorbed and authority is delegated to those in contact with 'reality'). For example, this was seen in the way that commissioners provided helpful information about other services, linked the new team to other key stakeholders, and provided networking opportunities to facilitate thinking and discussions. In thinking about leadership and management in personality disorder services, it would appear important for the leader to model tolerating ambiguity, managing power and authority, to know the detail and hold the big picture, and to be open and yet buffer the team. In addition, it became clear that leadership and management in personality disorder services is much more about judgement and balancing dialectics—for example, transparency versus holding anxiety, and modelling healthy coping and behaviour—far more than in traditional management where there can be absolutes and a final truth. For example, the lack of emphasis on the diagnostic approach (appropriate to this age group) led to a case formulation approach which provides a solid and shared understanding of a young man's difficulties. However, there were certainly some staff who wanted the clarity and certainty of shared language and understanding that comes with a diagnosis and were not so able to access the value of a case formulation approach.

As mentioned in the Introduction to the chapter, it is to be expected that there will be hurdles along the way to achieving integrated working and this is likely to continue to be the case as the service is delivered. These have revolved around trying to align health and prison service approaches and their expectation of approach, success, and meaningful involvement. This has also presented itself at times in the multi-disciplinary team (MDT).

If the primary task for the service design team was to focus on achieving the programme outcomes—that is, public protection, psychological health improvements, workforce development, and the effective use of resources—then the obvious hurdles were to be able to hold all of those in mind and ensure a service design and mix of staff who can work to all those outcomes. Experience and theoretical literature (see [30]) suggest that staff groups sometime interlock around the care versus control axis and in doing so can exploit the anxiety of the other. For example, when prisoners disclose information relevant to their risk in the future that was previously not known by those working with the prisoner, at what point should that information be passed on in the usual way to the security and offender management teams or how long can it be held between the OPD worker and the young man in order to maintain rapport and to contain the likely anxiety? Such forces need recognizing and managing so that any system or team does not become stale and closed but remains healthy and integrated with reality. Livesley's [31] work on the value of and approach to integrated treatment with this client group wholly supports this, as well as commenting particularly on the challenge to integrate treatment and security requirements in services.

At times, there were discussions in the MDT around how important status and hierarchy is in the context of a young adult male service where both of these are significant in the service users' lives. It also seemed that the age of the population drew more on the usual MDT dilemma of how to use a shared thinking space: the young men tend to demand action and resolution, and not delays while people think before acting. For example, when such young men experience anxiety and lack of containment, they often push those close to them to contain them and this can present in the prison environment as demanding transfers or threats to harm themselves or others to get moved out of their current location. This can nudge workers into knee-jerk reactions and taking responsibility from the young man in order to preserve safety. It is safe to say that no MDT arrives fully formed and able to use a shared space, to get straight to exploring personal responses and vulnerabilities in the work, so as to make use of the personal without it becoming personal. It takes time and support to arrive at that place for such thinking to be done. The aim though is always to try to hold the 'both/and' position, instead of the false dilemma of 'either/or' which sometimes gets adopted in MDTs and especially those working with challenging populations. The challenge for any team then is to find a way to work through the perspectives and experiences of the service user and the team while staying positive, collaborative, relational, and on track with the primary task.

A further challenge is the ongoing one when working with the age range being discussed here. In particular are the ethical issues that present when working with young adults who, while legally adult, are often immature emotionally and cognitively, and/or have low intellectual capacity, brain injury, substance-use issues, trauma, neglect in the family history, and a broken system of adults and caregivers before custody. To expect such a young person to be able to give informed consent is naïve, yet to ignore their wishes is not legal or ethical. The constant balance of that dilemma is present in such working, and more pointed in a service looking at emerging personality difficulties, where there is little clarity yet always a need for defensible and transparent practice—all this to consider when the population for the service are all in 'emerging adulthood' (see [32]) where developmental challenges and ongoing changes are the norm.

A key part of the service design was the need to embed a functional service user perspective. This approach in the early stages was informed by the service user literature in aiming to develop a service with the support of service user consultants as employed members of staff. It is important to ground service development in an appreciation of service user needs, their contribution, and how to develop them as leaders. Service users have direct experience of the way that services impact on their lives and so are best placed to comment on what works for them and what does not. This has been a particularly challenging aspect of the work in the context of a YOI that was only starting to adjust to doing meaningful service user involvement but was still resistant to what in the NHS would often be commonly accepted principles. Meaningful service user involvement in the custodial context will probably always bring dispute over power and hierarchy (see [33]). Issues of public protection and security may complicate service user involvement, although they are not reason enough to not seek to involve people. However, the practical implications of involving service users need to be addressed to ensure involvement is not tokenistic and does not seek to ignore difference for the more harmonious approach of concentrating on sameness.

In discussing what has worked well or not so well with regard to integrated working in OPD service design, the question is whether the same would be said about any service or whether there was something unique or emphasized in the OPD service in the context of young adult men in custody. For example, there is always room for improvement in the service's approach to ensuring the offer to the young men is tailored as closely as possible to their needs, age, and developmental stage when considering sequencing and tailoring interventions to their readiness to engage. When services succeed in this regard it seems that the adolescent features of this age group are held in mind but do not present an insurmountable barrier to treatment; for example, the YOI team is able to respond to fluctuating motivation with patience and consistency.

The particular service in question has succeeded so far in offering a creative approach to the services being offered in a custodial setting, with a service design that offers assertive outreach across the prison as well as interventions offered in a dedicated space for a range of psychological and occupational art, drama, and music therapies. It has already been recognized that any mental health or well-being service needs to be able to respond to the diversity of ethnicities and identities in its population, and the YOI OPD service is no exception. Work is ongoing to ensure that engagement activities and therapeutic tools are as culturally responsive and competent as they should be to respond to a population roughly half white and half black and minority ethnic in its make-up.

The governance team has worked constantly through the various issues arising with recruitment and retention to ensure the team is still well balanced in terms of skills and health or justice staff. It was sometimes difficult to source the suitably skilled people and agencies to provide the required service: for example, art therapists, systemic therapists, and forensic psychologists. Balance in the model is crucial to ensure the care versus control axis is stable and the team mind is refracted through the lens of various perspectives. For example, a justice-dominant team can tend to focus more on the perpetrator aspect of the prisoner and his or her experience, without fully taking account of how victim experiences link in. Similarly, a health-dominant team can sometimes underestimate or misunderstand the presenting risks and/or custodial setting, which does little to offer containment and understanding to the service user, or progress towards release.

What stands out in terms of where the service is now and the challenges for it going forward is how well it will respond to the usual ebb and flow of projections and defences in the wider prison that will seek perhaps to reject or project into the reflective and relational way of working. That can present as the wider staff team in the prison begrudging the unique way in which staff within the OPD team are able to work with the young men and so accuse them of 'molly coddling', or not wanting to do usual operational work in the prison, or of being blind to what the prisoner 'is really like'. Ensuring an understanding of the nature and complexity of the task is important in keeping the service fully integrated into the wider setting when this happens. The focus on integrated working is not just between commissioners, health, and prison service staff, but integrating prisoners all the way through the offender pathways, whether into their next placement—be that another OPD service or an adult jail—integrating them back into their family, or ultimately integrating them back into the community. If integrated working is the focus, it should bring together a system where each part is valuable in itself but part of a single totality that is even more valuable as a whole.

The experience in probation

Many of the challenges described in jointly developing and delivering OPD services in secure settings are also relevant to OPD services in the community. Here, the key relationship is between NHS-employed psychologists and HMPPS-employed offender managers. The nature of this relationship is influenced by a number of factors, not least the lead role of the offender manager in overseeing individuals' progression through their sentence and the significant organizational changes within probation since the inception of the OPD pathway.

By 2010, a London mental health trust working with the probation service in London developed and successfully implemented the Personality Disorder Pilot Project in a few local areas within the London probation area. This project was set up to work with people with complex personality issues and high harm behaviours using probation officers and NHS psychologists to identify traits of personality disorder. The objective was to assist probation staff in working with and understanding the issues of personality disorder in managing risks posed by this group of offenders. The project aimed to develop, pilot, and test a pathway that would enhance the effective management of these offenders and ensure their early identification, to provide high-quality assessments to assist the court and support sentence planning, ensuring that interventions are appropriately planned and psychologically informed.

This pilot project was developed using grant funding, but from July 2010 secured continuation funding from the Department of Health/NOMS DSPD programme which in various forms continued until the contracts for the Community Pathway were let in April 2013. The new contract created a formal working relationship with a wider range of health partners (four London NHS trusts) who came together in a consortium. Probation officers had a role in delivering the service within the contract and were recruited to work alongside the NHS psychologists. The new Community Pathway was now commissioned and working to a service specification which was building on the good foundation of the pilot.

In May 2014, under government policy of Transforming Rehabilitation (TR), Probation Trusts were abolished, resulting in the division of probation caseloads into two cohorts: the new NPS took high-risk, serious offenders, all MAPPA cases and all Foreign Offender cases retaining their management in the public sector; medium- and low-risk cases were allocated to a host of private organizations generally termed Community Rehabilitation Companies (CRCs).

In London it was possible to ensure that all probation officers working on the pathway would remain in the public sector and transfer to the NPS, and since the cases screened in were in the higher-risk categories, these also transferred to the NPS, ensuring that community pathway services were sustained throughout this period of major change.

The former Probation Trust staff group was split between these two organizations, with an acknowledged high level of anxiety in staff in both the new organizations [34] and a need to adjust to new systems, processes, and management. The Audit Commission reviewed the impact of TR and reported that the NPS had higher than predicted caseloads and faced significant understaffing, with some staff working at more than 125% capacity. NPS frontline managers (Senior Probation Officers (SPOs)) faced increasing pressure, including dealing with the higher than expected workloads of high-risk offenders, while assimilating an unexpectedly heavy influx of trainees to meet the staff shortage. At the same time, probation managers in the NPS were acquiring new responsibilities for managing support services, such as human resources and office management. A major impact of this has been that staff supervision was either not delivered or, when it was, the supervision focused on performance measures rather than improving the quality of work delivered [35]. Middle managers (SPOs) should be key to the implementation of a program such as the OPD pathway, ensuring local integration into offender management and by creating both the learning environment for this work and the physical environment for delivery. This continues to be a weakness in pathway delivery.

Additionally, both managers and frontline staff have had to cope with laborious and dated computerized case and offender management systems which have not been supportive of the ambitions of the Community Pathway.

In November 2015, the NPS introduced a further national change programme [36] to tackle regional variations in delivery and to develop the NPS as an effective, efficient, and excellent service. Therefore, there is the risk that staff 'change fatigue' may continue into the future and it will be some time before these weaknesses can be addressed.

Despite system turbulence, the implementation and delivery of the OPD pathway in the community in London continues and is generally welcomed by staff, who can now clearly see the benefit that the Community Pathway brings to both offenders and probation officers in engaging this difficult and needy offender group.

The role of the commissioners in bedding in this project has been notably positive. It is highly appropriate that in a pathway that is *relational* the commissioners model this behaviour. In the London Community Personality Disorder Pathway, both at development and implementation, the commissioners have been committed to a leadership ethos, modelled and promoted collaborative working, demonstrated flexibility, and supported innovation. They were crucial in establishing a genuine partnership approach, which can often be difficult in a contractual relationship, and have ensured total commitment to the underpinning philosophy of the pathway which is joint responsibility at co-commissioning and service delivery level.

The delivery environment for the OPD pathway in London is complex and developing, covering thirty three London boroughs and, as has been described above, has been beset with change since the beginning of the contract. Despite the enormity of this restructure and the challenges posed, the pathway continued to be supported and promoted by London Division senior management, and the main elements of the pathway remained operational, meeting the required key performance indicators (KPIs). This was testimony to the robustness of the partnership arrangements developed and a commitment to the philosophy of joint delivery.

Despite strong leadership, particularly from commissioners, and having a partnership that has robustly stood rigorous testing, there are many challenges with a service of this nature in a complex regional setting.

There are knowledge and cultural differences between health and criminal justice providers. In terms of the knowledge base, as would be expected, generally the probation staff have a greater understanding of the operation of the criminal justice system and the priorities of that system around reducing further offending and managing risk. They have a working knowledge of the Courts, the Parole System, and MAPPAs. They have been trained in enforcement and have a commitment to rehabilitation and an understanding of desistance. They have to work with the very real tensions in balancing individuals' rights and their need to challenge and test on the way to change with the wider protection of the public and victims alongside the adherence to court orders and licence conditions. Probation staff understand confidentiality in a risk context and have a commitment to robust information exchange with partners to promote public protection.

This compares with health staff who have much more clinical knowledge and practice around managing personality disorder and other behaviours, and have a better understanding of individuals' developmental histories and the impact on their personalities and maladaptive behaviours. The rules governing confidentiality and the impact, both on patient and practitioner, of disclosure are very different to those experienced by criminal justice service colleagues, and generally the health commitment to recovery and patient self-determination can generate a different approach to disclosure than that expected within the probation environment.

There is also an issue of professional confidence that comes with health partners who often feel that they must be in control as experts and should automatically be in a lead position. However, in the criminal justice service environment it is essential to understand that the probation officer is the case owner, and all provision delivered by the pathway supports the probation office in this role and supports the officer in helping to identify issues relating to potential personality difficulties and better understand the offender.

There are obvious advantages of this amalgamation of knowledge and indeed it is key to shared responsibility and joint operations, but the cultural differences, if not addressed and corrected for, might interfere with maximizing the opportunity to work as one in addressing risk, reducing reoffending, and promoting well-being.

Likewise with communication; if clear and open communication is not a priority and central to operations then there is a risk of compounding the cultural difficulties and possibly creating splitting within the staff groups. Communication issues arise from several sources, including the challenge of working with a large workforce, use of different IT systems, and line management structures that are outside the project.

Performance is another area that has proved challenging and requires collaborative management to effect the joint responsibility principle of the OPD pathway.

The pathway delivery includes a mix of professions, including clinical and forensic psychologists at various grades and probation officers. Jointly these staff should work with probation to identify cases with features of personality difficulty, to provide consultation and formulation, and to focus on probation staff development and training. In a few most difficult, limited cases, pathway staff may also do some joint caseworking. It is also desirable that the pathway identifies creative responses to difficulties identified in working with a personality disorder cohort.

Performance generally will be measured against KPIs, but other measures may also need to be considered. If poor performance is identified it can be a challenge to pinpoint and assess the causes, but an overemphasis on managerial KPIs can create pressure on data recording, impact negatively on staff morale, and be counterproductive in terms of project impact. Having clearly defined tasks and roles can assist in monitoring individual performance. Such an approach would need to include defining the role of the operational SPO who has responsibility for line management of the pathway probation officers and for their personal development and annual appraisal.

It is essential that the pathway is integrated into NPS practice and not be considered a special project or add-on. The pathway is core to the operational needs of the NPS and the working agreement between the agencies needs to reflect this. It is also important that any national change programme understands that pathway work is offender management and that any change made to the operating model could have a major impact on the pathway effectiveness if not built into the change.

To develop, this project needs to demonstrate, and is working on demonstrating, the impact on offenders and probation staff. It needs to be able to show that it is not simply an add-on, but that it is offender management, albeit that it brings added value to offender management, as was, prior to the implementation of the OPD pathway. It must be able to demonstrate that it makes a difference; to do this requires continued cooperation with commissioners and that these people are able to think outside the box, and not to be totally driven by restrictive KPIs.

Partnership is pivotal to joint delivery and to better outcomes for offenders with personality disorder. A genuine partnership is one that is not essentially target driven but is a way of working based on a can-do approach that is aimed at reducing inequalities for its service users. It must transcend individual practitioners, for the pathway must embrace the underpinning set of values.

Senior and Kinsella [37], in their review of a long-term criminal justice partnership in London, state that effective partnership should have the capacity to open doors and to garner expertise. This research suggests three key features to effective partnership:

- Joint and consistent leadership
- Flexible and diverse use of funds
- Modelling good practice approaches.

The OPD pathway in the community in London has many of the features of good partnership, and indeed many of the problems generated in this pathway are a result of a blurring of the boundaries of the agencies—almost a problem of success.

Concluding remarks

Our overall conclusion is that co-commissioning has been a striking success, albeit associated with some tensions in partnership working. This has been achieved with committed leadership - from commissioners, within LPP's steering group, and from our probation and prison partners-and this will be tested as key personnel change. The robustness of the organisational relationships will be proven by their capacity to manage challenges without reverting to former ways of working.

References

1. **Department of Health, Ministry of Justice**. Consultation on the Offender Personality Disorder pathway implementation plan. Leeds: Department of Health; 2011. http://cipn. org.uk/wp-content/uploads/2017/05/personality_disorder_pathway_feb_11.pdf.

2. **Livesley WJ.** An integrated approach to the treatment of personality disorder. Journal of Mental Health. 2007;**16**(1):131–148.

3. **National Report for the National Co-ordinating Centre for NHS Service Delivery and Organisation R&D (NCCSDO).** Learning the lessons: a multimethod evaluation of dedicated community-based services for people with personality disorder. London: HMSO; 2007.

4. **Cardona OD.** Environmental management and disaster prevention: two related topics: a holistic risk assessment and management approach. In J Ingleton (Ed.), Natural disaster management. London: Tudor Rose; 1999, pp. 151–153.

5. **Menzies Lyth I.** Containing anxiety in institutions, Vol. 1. London: Free Association Books; 1988.

6. **Bradley KJ.** The Bradley Report: Lord Bradley's review of people with mental health problems or learning disabilities in the criminal justice system. London: Department of Health; 2009.

7. **Secretaries of State for Health, Wales, Northern Ireland and Scotland.** Working for patients. Cm 555. London: HMSO; 1989.

8. **Department of Health.** The new NHS: modern, dependable. London: Department of Health; 1997.

9. **Department of Health.** The NHS plan: a plan for investment, a plan for reform. London: The Stationery Office; 2000.

10. **Carter P.** Managing offenders, reducing crime: a new approach. London: Home Office Strategy Unit; 2003.

11. **Department of Health.** Health and Social Care Act. London: The Stationery Office; 2012.

12. **Dowler C.** Hunt interview: CQC ratings have replaced FT status as 'definition of success'. Local Government Chronicle; 9 September 2015. https://www.lgcplus.com/ services/health-and-care/hunt-interview-cqc-ratings-have-replaced-ft-status-as-definition-of-success/5090190.article.

13. **NHS England.** The forward view into action: planning for 2015/16. Leeds: NHS England; 2014.

14. **Davies P.** Your shout: interview with Mark Britnell. In View. 2007;**15**(3).

15. **Britnell M.** 'Commission impossible'? Is world class commissioning achievable in the NHS? Debate hosted by Civitas, Grand Committee Room, House of Commons, London, 16 July 2008.

16. **Woodin J, Wade E.** Towards world class commissioning competency. Birmingham: University of Birmingham; 2007.

17. **European Foundation for the Improvement of Living and Working Conditions.** European Quality of Life Survey. Loughlinstown: European Foundation for the Improvement of Living and Working Conditions; 2003.

18. **Coomans G.** Europe's changing demography: constraints and bottlenecks. Demographic and social trends issue paper, No. 8. Seville: Joint Research Centre (JRC), and Institute for Prospective Technological Studies (IPTS); 1999.

19. **NHS Institute for Innovation and Improvement.** Commissioning to make a bigger difference. A guide for NHS and social care commissioners on promoting service innovation. London: HMSO; 2008.

20. **Department of Health.** World class commissioning. Vision. London: HMSO; 2007.

21. **Department of Health.** Response to the offender personality disorder consultation. London: Department of Health; 2011.

22. **National Offender Management Service, Department of Health.** Working with personality disordered offenders: a practitioner's guide. London: National Offender Management Service, and Department of Health; 2011.

23. **Royal College of Psychiatrists.** Enabling Environment standards. London: Royal College of Psychiatrists; 2013.

24. **Stokoe P.** The healthy and the unhealthy organisation: how can we help teams to remain effective? In A Rubitel and D Reiss (Eds.), In the community: frameworks for thinking about antisocial behaviour and mental health. London: Karnac Books; 2011, pp. 237–259.

25. **Kahn WA.** Holding fast: the struggle to create resilient caregiving organisations. Hove: Brunner-Routledge; 2005.

26. **Price K, Gillespie S, Rutter D, Dhillon K, Gibson S, Faulkner A, Weaver T, Crawford MJ.** Dedicated personality disorder services: a qualitative analysis of service structure and treatment process. Journal of Mental Health. 2009;**18**(6):467–475.

27. **Bion W.** Experiences in groups. London: Tavistock; 1961.

28. **Roth A, Pilling, S.** A competence framework for psychological interventions with people with personality disorder. www.ucl.ac.uk/pals/research/clinical-educational-and-health-psychology/research-groups/core/competence-frameworks-12.

29. **Obholzer A.** The leader, the unconscious, and the management of the organization. In LJ Gould, LF Stapley, and M Stein (Eds.), The systems psychodynamics of organizations: integrating the group relations approach, psychoanalytic, and open systems perspectives. London: Karnac Books; 2001, pp. 197–216.

30. **Skogstad W.** Internal and external reality: enquiring into their interplay in an inpatient setting. In L Day and P Pringle (Eds.), Reflective enquiry into therapeutic institutions. London: Karnac Books; 2001, pp. 45–65.

31. **Livesley WJ, Dimaggio G, Clarkin JF.** Integrated treatment for personality disorder. London: Guildford Press; 2016.

32. **Arnett JJ.** Adolescence and emerging adulthood: a cultural approach, 3rd edn. Upper Saddle River, NJ: Prentice Hall; 2007.

33. **Crawford M.** Involving users in the development of psychiatric services—no longer an option. Psychiatric Bulletin. 2001;**25**:84–86.

34. **National Audit Office.** Transforming rehabilitation. London: Ministry of Justice; 2016.

35. **HM Inspectorate of Probation.** Transforming Rehabilitation: early implementation 5. Manchester: HM Inspectorate of Probation; 2016.

36. **National Probation Service.** NPS operating model: effective, efficient, excellent. London: HM Prison Service; 2016.

37. **Senior P, Kinsella R.** A working partnership: an analysis of the relationship between probation in London and Together for Mental Wellbeing. Sheffield: Hallam Centre for Community Justice; 2014.

Chapter 8

Making an impact: Have we got it right yet?

Jackie Craissati and Colin Campbell

Introduction

This is an opportunity for the editors—with unapologetic subjectivity—to look back at the preceding chapters and reflect on the achievements and learning from the past few years. It seems impossible not to conclude that, overall, the changes in delivery of services to personality disordered offenders over the past decade have been hugely beneficial. We have made progress in so many ways: building a motivated and increasingly skilled workforce; designing a 'good enough' screening process which does not require specialist expertise; and driving a model of formulation-based delivery, whether it be consultation, therapy, or psychologically informed management. Most astonishing of all, we appear to have achieved this in a largely consistent and coherent way across England and Wales, with joint operations from criminal justice and health providers at a time of unprecedented economic pressure and scrutiny of our public services. The London Pathways Partnership (LPP) has been at the heart of these developments, and we are justifiably proud of the contribution we have made to the national picture.

So why worry so much about impact, about the question of whether we are making a difference that really adds value? Impact matters because we are spending many millions of pounds of public money to work with a group of individuals—albeit seriously disabled by their psychological difficulties—who have inflicted harm on others and may well pose a high risk of doing so again if in the community. The money needs to be spent wisely, and the benefits to everyone—the public and the offender—explicitly demonstrated. This is no mean task, and in the section 'Evaluation of the OPD strategy' we highlight some of the complexities of evidencing impact by means of research. There are also considerable dangers inherent in complacency—'We have done well, better than before, we believe in what we are doing, so why question it?'—so we need to find our critical friends, and use them to keep one step ahead; many services have floundered by failing to review and revise their product.

The OPD strategy has, at its heart, a focus on formulation as the driver for conceptualizing individual offender difficulties. We felt it would be appropriate to adopt the same formulation-based approach to appraising our progression to this point in time; most importantly, we wanted to explore the assumptions and drivers for change associated with each key stage of the process in the past ten years.

The presenting problem

In using a formulation-based approach it is essential that the presenting problem is clearly defined, understood, and shared between the relevant stakeholders, since we know that the most effective personality disorder services have coherent and explicit models of care to which all stakeholders sign up. In relation to the OPD strategy, there are three key stakeholders. First, there are the *funders*—the government—which have a political agenda and which both represent and are accountable to the electorate. Second, there are the *providers*, who come from a range of criminal justice and health professional backgrounds, with accompanying agendas in relation to expertise, responsibility, professional codes of conduct, and ethics. Third, there are the *recipients*—personality disordered offenders, who are burdened with their personal experiences which colour their world view, and who may not always act in their own best interests. We conceptualize the commissioners as acting as a 'broker' between each of these key stakeholders (see Fig. 8.1).

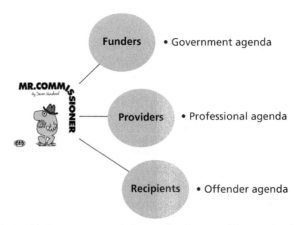

Fig. 8.1 Relationship between commissioners, funders, providers, and recipients

The assumption that the three stakeholders in this model agree on the presenting problem and the formulation that underpins it needs to be challenged, and we do so here in relation to both the DSPD programme and the OPD pathway model.

DSPD: the first provisional hypothesis

The presenting problem—as conceptualized by the DSPD programme—was that there were '500 [of the] most dangerous men in the country' who were personality disordered and not currently able to access treatment. This assumption was predicated on an illness model [1]. That is, the focus of the programme was a diagnosis, which was treated largely by health professionals (or those with psychological training) using a biopsychological 'expert' model in specialist, stand-alone services (see Table 8.1).

Eligibility for the services required a diagnosis of not only personality disorder but also 'severe' personality disorder, variously defined as diagnoses from within multiple clusters of personality disorders or a particular score on the Psychopathy Checklist–Revised (PCL-R). There were also stringent risk criteria, such that the services would only consider those who posed the highest risk of harm to others. Consistent with an illness model, there was a strong emphasis on diagnosis, meticulously achieved with an extensive minimum dataset of personality and risk assessments. The intention of the services was to deliver

Table 8.1 Illness model

Focus	Symptom; diagnosis; illness; impairment
	Absence of disease or disability
	Disease centred
Evidence base	Biomedical
	Does not take into consideration wider influences on health
	Scientific
	Expert model
Input	Doctor; health professional
Approach	Assessment, monitoring, programme of intervention imposed
	Segregation and alternative services
	Ordinary needs put on hold
	Individual is faulty
	Individual is passive and doctor fixes the condition
	Individual is passive recipient of treatment
	Individual has personal responsibility for health
	Problem is a feature of the person, not of society
	Problem is something to be cured

treatment with an intensity that matched the severity of the condition; this was often imposed on the patient who often either was a passive recipient or actively resisted engaging in treatment. Treatment was largely delivered in high-secure institutions, partly due to the focus on those posing the highest risk, but undoubtedly with societal concerns about risk at the time in mind, too.

The successes and failures of the DSPD programme have been summarized elsewhere (see Chapter 1). We suggest that one of the reasons for the programme difficulties was the disparity in the working hypotheses of the key stakeholders (Fig. 8.2). From the *funders'* perspective, the aim of the DSPD services was to keep high-risk offenders detained and, in doing so, protect the public. It is reasonable to assume that the public agreed that the government should fund humane containment and access to treatment for these offenders; it is less clear that the public were committed to such offenders returning to their communities eventually. Success, in terms of risk reduction, was never explicitly defined, and the implication was that a zero-violent reoffending rate was the only acceptable outcome. The upshot was that only a handful of offenders benefited and there was little movement back to the community. There was no evidence of a broader impact on rates of sexual or violent reoffending—much less the desired 'zero' reoffending—and the services were not cost-effective.

From the *providers'* perspective, one of the key successes was the development of a skilled workforce, primarily in health but also in the criminal justice system. However, this was limited to isolated centres of best practice, each developing their own centre of excellence without reference to each other or the wider public sector. In other aspects, the agendas of health and criminal justice differed slightly. Initial enthusiasm by health providers was often replaced by the anxiety associated with the everyday management of a complex high-risk

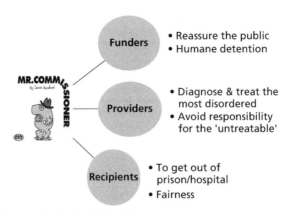

Fig. 8.2 DSPD organizational relationships

patient group and a concern to avoid organizational risk. Providers developed a range of clinically oriented treatment approaches, which had an impact primarily on psychological well-being, with public protection very much a secondary aim. There were also significant ethical concerns in detaining an aggrieved population of patients transferred from prison close to their end of sentence, who failed to engage in treatment, creating concerns about them simply being 'warehoused'. In contrast, criminal justice services were content to receive the additional resources to manage personality disordered offenders who were already an existing responsibility for them.

In many ways, the *recipients* of DSPD services were caught between the contrasting agendas of the funders and providers. A small number of recipients clearly had access to treatment that they would not have had prior to the DSPD programme, but the majority of high-risk offenders with personality disorder were excluded from the programme. Expectations of just or fair treatment are likely to have been undermined, not only by transfer to hospital close to the end of sentence, when prisoners were anticipating release, but also by a more pervasive problem that almost all treatment opportunities were linked with a possible extension of detention of around five to ten years. The perception that engaging in treatment had become the only way to progress towards release undermined collaboration in treatment and had a negative impact on motivation to engage. The perception that engaging in treatment was a necessary prerequisite of a successful Parole Board hearing could have a similar effect. The not uncommon endpoint of aggrieved disengagement—deselection—was also a powerful obstacle to progression, particularly if combined with a high PCL-R score, which precluded access to most offending behaviour programmes.

The OPD pathway: revising the provisional hypothesis

We would postulate that the OPD pathway strategy represented a move away from an illness model towards a public health model. Table 8.2 outlines the elements of a public health model which can be contrasted with the illness model outlined in Table 8.1. That is, public health models take a population and prevention approach rather than an individual and diagnosis-focused approach; the emphasis is on human behaviour, health promotion, and environmental interventions [2]. This contrasts with the treatment and medical care approach of the illness model.

Although the OPD strategy has restricted itself to personality disordered offenders, it could be argued that the focus has been a total population approach in terms of offenders. Within these constraints, the OPD pathway has delivered a public health intervention at the primary, secondary, and tertiary levels, as shown in Fig. 8.3. This public health model reflects the OPD strategy's shift to

Table 8.2 Public health model

Focus	Health/safety/well-being of entire populations Maximum benefit for the largest number of people Seeks to improve the health and safety of all individuals by addressing underlying risk factors that increase the likelihood that an individual will become a victim or a perpetrator of violence Primary prevention of violence by exposing a broad segment of a population to prevention measures and to reduce and prevent violence at a population level
Evidence base	Multi-disciplinary, broad knowledge base Medicine, epidemiology, sociology, psychology, criminology, education, economics
Input	Diverse sectors Health, education, social services, justice, policy, private sector
Approach	Rooted in scientific method 1. Define/monitor the problem—magnitude—who/what/where/when/how. To define the problem through the systematic collection of information about the magnitude, scope, characteristics, and consequences of violence 2. Identify risk and protective factors—help identify where prevention efforts need to be focused. To establish why violence occurs using research to determine the causes and correlates of violence, the factors that increase or decrease the risk for violence, and the factors that could be modified through interventions 3. Develop and test prevention strategies—based on research literature, needs assessments, community surveys, stakeholder interviews, focus groups—then rigorously evaluated. To find out what works to prevent violence by designing, implementing, and evaluating interventions 4. Assure widespread adoption—training, networking, technical assistance—evaluation. To implement effective and promising interventions in a wide range of settings. The effects of these interventions on risk factors and the target outcome should be monitored, and their impact and cost-effectiveness should be evaluated

a psycho-educational approach to non-specialist staff, the focus on more responsive environments and replacing the emphasis on diagnosis and specialist treatments with a predominant focus on broader concepts of psychological dysfunction and management approaches embedded in everyday service provision.

Although not without its difficulties and limitations, it is arguable that the premise on which the OPD strategy is based is more aligned when considering the perspective of funders, providers, and recipients. That is, there is a revised formulation to which all three stakeholders have now been able to subscribe

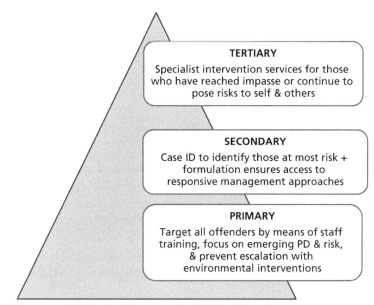

Fig. 8.3 Levels of public health intervention for the OPD pathway

in a more coherent fashion. *Funders* have committed to joint operations be-tween criminal justice and mental health, at all levels of delivery, with the aim of improving outcomes for all personality disordered offenders; importantly, the strategy explicitly states the need for the criminal justice system to take primary responsibility for its offenders, and that delivery begins and ends with the community perspective. *Providers* have delivered within this overarching structure, adhering to a single psychologically informed approach to the man-agement of offenders with *pervasive psychological difficulties. Recipients*—no longer just the offenders, but also the frontline staff most frequently working with the offenders—have access to a more-responsive range of less-specialist options with improved perceptions of 'fairness'.

This shared formulation regarding the principles of the OPD pathway has led to coherent and consistent service delivery. However, as the preceding chap-ters have highlighted, this has not been without its problems. For example, unanticipated political change has almost 'derailed' the strategy, and these re-visions to public service delivery are likely to emerge again in the near future. Partnership working has not been without its tensions, and it is undoubtedly easier to slip back into working in parallel rather than in integrated partner-ships; workforce limitations and organizational imperatives regularly interfere with the principles of joint delivery, drawing practitioners back into habitual ways of working. Practitioners find it difficult not to become preoccupied with their own aspect of the pathway—whether in the community or a secure institution—and this tendency to look inwards and remain in the here and now has to be constantly challenged; a pathway approach requires practitioners and services to hold in mind where the offender has come from and where he/she is heading.

Evaluation of the OPD strategy

If we now return to the question posed at the start of this chapter: that is, does the OPD pathway strategy make a difference in terms of the impact on the high-level outcomes? Can we go beyond the question of service quality—so often confused with questions of service outcomes—and ask ourselves whether the new strategy has diluted resources to such an extent that it has compromised our ability to have a discernible impact?

Research and evaluation is embedded in the OPD strategy, as it was in the DSPD programme. However, evaluating such a complex network of services presents several challenges:

- Commissioning evaluation of OPD services needs to take into consideration the multiple aims of the pathway, including reducing reoffending, improving psychological well-being, and efficient use of resources. Evaluation assumes that these multiple processes, outcomes, and impacts are somehow inter-related and that not only are the interventions involved lengthy, but also the related outcomes require a significant follow-up period to be reliably identified. Therefore, any evaluation requires not only a detailed understanding of the services and how they work but also an innovative multi-method approach to investigating a diverse range of outcomes. Failure to do this can limit the utility of well-executed research. For example, one of the 'headlines' of the DSPD evaluation was that patients in these expensive services were having less than two hours a week of face-to-face therapy [3]. However, given that many of these patients had been transferred to these services shortly before their sentence expired and that many had never engaged in treatment before, it is perhaps unsurprising that many were aggrieved and unmotivated and therefore unlikely to engage in intensive treatment. This finding also does not preclude the possibility that, having completed some initial motivational work and engaged in various aspects of the therapeutic environment, such patients would go on to successfully engage in treatment. Limited resources also meant that the follow-up period was unlikely to detect whether or not this happened, much less what the impact was on, arguably, the primary aim of these services, which was to reduce risk and reoffending.

- Understandably, at the outset of such major programmes, developing extensive databases can seem like an opportunity too good to be missed. However, these databases are only as good as the data entered into them and a number of factors have limited their success in evaluation of services for offenders with personality disorder. Focusing on delivering a safe, effective clinical service can be a powerful distraction from routine data collection, particularly if the data in question are not perceived as obviously related to delivering such a service. The fundamental problem is that the data needed to provide the service are not always the same as those needed to evaluate it. Staff working in these demanding services are always going to be reluctant to record data they don't need or can't see the point of and this needs to be understood from a systemic, organizational perspective, in addition to any more practical approaches to the problem.

- A related problem is that relevant routinely collected data are often held in multiple databases across the health and criminal justice services. The lack of common identifiers across these databases significantly restricts opportunities to link data and therefore the utility of large-scale evaluations investigating multiple health and criminal justice outcomes. The slightly bigger question is whether, even with effective data collection, data linking, and multi-method approaches, it is possible to effectively evaluate complex constructs such as managing transitions, the timing and sequencing of interventions, effective collaboration, and the impact of therapeutic environments, which may be central to the success of individual offender's pathways.

In the light of the above difficulties, there has been an important role within the OPD pathway implementation for locally devised and implemented evaluation projects. Although methodologically less robust, these projects have been driven by practitioner interest and a commitment to achieving best practice; they have resulted in more immediate opportunities for reflection and review.

Below we summarize our state of knowledge regarding the pathway and the four high-level outcomes.

To reduce sexual/violent reoffending

Although we have some indication that pathway interventions may have reduced criminogenic need in personality disordered offenders participating in services, these data are not consistent [4], and we do not have definitive recidivism data. The early pilots identified that participating offenders were less likely to fail in the community [5, 6], but we do not know if this was a causal relationship.

To improve offender well-being

This outcome has been seriously hampered by a lack of clarity and definition as to what 'well-being' comprises. Thus far, we have some qualitative data on offender satisfaction and some environmental and therapeutic alliance data [7], all of which are cautiously positive. However, in terms of positive changes in psychological functioning and emotional stability—if that is how we wish to define well-being—no clear findings have been established.

To improve workforce competence and confidence

This is perhaps the outcome most robustly evaluated, with the most consistent findings (e.g. [8, 9]). That is, we could evidence improved competence and confidence in the workforce as a result of both training and consultancy (these two aspects often being undifferentiated in the research methodology). We are beginning to demonstrate that non-specialist non-mental health professionals can adopt a formulation-based approach. However, we do not, as yet, know whether such improvements are translated into enhanced skills when working with offenders, and whether these enhanced skills lead to other positive outcomes.

To deploy limited resources efficiently

It may seem self-evident that the OPD strategy uses limited resources more efficiently, in terms of spread and access. The key, however, rests with an economic evaluation of the impact of the strategy in terms of cost weighed up against benefit, and we will need to wait for this analysis.

Summary: reworking the formulation to understand the mechanism of change

In considering next steps, our view is that the OPD pathway strategy has largely been a success, with emerging evidence to offer some support for influencing outcomes. It is clear that we now have a strategy for personality disordered offenders which has greatly increased accessibility, thereby providing a more economically viable service which is arguably fairer for the recipients. The strategy is not without its areas of weakness, as we have pointed out, perhaps the most pressing of which is the uncertainty regarding its impact on future sexual and violent reoffending rates, and the lack of rigour in considering the nature and role of psychological well-being in the model. In other words, have we spread our aims and resources so thin that our potential to change hard outcomes has diminished?

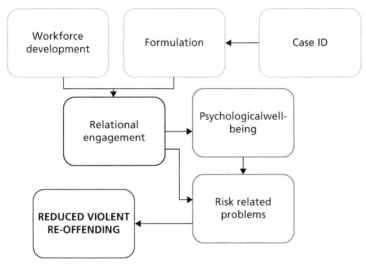

Fig. 8.4 Model of change for the OPD pathway

It seems apposite to return to the theoretical underpinnings of the psychologically informed model adopted by the LPP, as described in Chapter 1. Our premise was that integrating ideas of attachment and desistence provided an evidence-based and accessible theoretical base for developing services. Within this integrated model—unapologetically community focused—our aim was to provide offenders with the opportunity to develop a new sense of a prosocial self, combined with a social investment in the community, achieved via a relational model. In essence, psychological well-being was conceptualized as relating to feeling understood by others in order to better understand oneself and, in doing so, achieve new ways of thinking about one's relationship to the world.

We would tentatively suggest that the aims and vision of the OPD pathway strategy are on the right lines, and there is no need to radically change the direction of travel. However, we do feel that a combination of gradually emerging evidence and clinical experience over the past three to four years suggests that the time has come to re-examine the high-level outcomes of the strategy and tighten our hypothesis as to the mechanism of change (or the means by which the strategy and its operationalization is likely to achieve the outcomes). Fig. 8.4 provides a figurative representation of our revised hypothesis.

The ultimate goal of the pathway is for high-risk violent offenders with pervasive psychological difficulties to be able to maximize their opportunities to lead an offence-free and reasonable quality of life in the community without placing the public at risk.

There are two core elements to the OPD pathway intervention that comprise the initial step to driving change within the model: first, *workforce development*; and second, a *formulation-based* approach. These two elements address the aspiration to deliver an *economically efficient* service:

♦ A cascade model for the dissemination of practitioner knowledge and skills has the ability to achieve a wider range of influence than a focus on specialist therapists implementing an expensive treatment approach.

♦ Case identification is simply a non-technical and accessible means of ensuring—at least to a reasonable extent—that the strategy deploys its limited resources on the right offenders; in many ways, this is a standardized triage approach. It allows a more targeted formulation-based management of the offender and drives a more focused sentence plan.

Our suggestion is that these two core elements have a direct impact on what we have called *relational engagement*. By this we mean the ability of the identified offender and the practitioner to think constructively and in collaboration, as a result of improved emotional containment, validation, and/or understanding.

We have not put consultation into the model, but this is not because we do not consider it a very important element of the strategy. The purpose of consultation—in our view—is primarily to develop and to communicate the formulation; that is, it is a process—a two-way process—but not a core driver within the model.

We would hypothesize that it is relational engagement that drives improvements in either *psychological well-being* or *reductions in risk-related problems*. Note that we do not think there is evidence to support a direct link between psychological well-being and reduced *violent reoffending* rates; we suggest that reductions in emotional distress and improved self-esteem create a context in which an offender is more able to 'mentalize'—in other words, to achieve the cognitive transformation and seek out the human and social capital necessary for desistance to take place. However, psychological well-being is not necessarily a prerequisite for reduced risk-related problems in our model, as we consider improved relational engagement can also have a direct relationship with reduced risk-related problems as levels of non-compliance and drop-out reduce and offenders can maximize the potential benefits of completed interventions.

The above model seems to more accurately reflect the current evidence base and clinical experience to date. We would argue that the tighter the formulation and the more it can be articulated and shared between all stakeholders, the more likely it is to be effective in terms of outcomes. Our future direction of travel in terms of evaluation will then need to reflect the model of change.

References

1. **Laing, R.** The politics of the family and other essays. London: Routledge; 1971.

2. **Mercy JA, Rosenberg ML, Powell KE, Broome CV, Roper WL.** Public health policy for preventing violence. Health Affairs. 1993;**12**:7–29.

3. **Trebilcock J, Weaver T.** Multi-method Evaluation of the Management, Organisation and Staffing (MEMOS) in high security treatment services for people with Dangerous and Severe Personality Disorder (DSPD). London: Ministry of Justice; 2010.

4. **Minoudis P, Kane E.** It's a journey, not a destination—from Dangerous and Severe Personality Disorder (DSPD) to the Offender Personality Disorder (OPD) pathway. Criminal Behaviour and Mental Health. 2017;**27**:207–213.

5. **Clark S, Chuan S.** Evaluation of the Impact Personality Disorder Project—a psychologically-informed consultation, training and mental health collaboration approach to probation offender management. Criminal Behaviour and Mental Health. 2015;**26**(3):186–195.

6. **Minoudis P, Shaw J, Craissati J.** The London Pathways Project: evaluating the effectiveness of a consultation model for personality disordered offenders. Criminal Behaviour and Mental Health. 2012;**22**:218–232.

7. **Shaw J, Higgins C, Quartey C.** The impact of collaborative case formulation with high risk offenders with personality disorder. Journal of Forensic Psychiatry & Psychology. 2017;**28**(6):777–789.

8. **Knauer V, Walker J, Roberts A.** Offender Personality Disorder pathway: the impact of case consultation and formulation with probation staff. Journal of Forensic Psychiatry & Psychology. 2017;**28**(6):825–840.

9. **Shaw J, Minoudis P, Craissati J, Bannerman A.** Developing probation staff competency for working with high risk of harm offenders with personality disorder: an evaluation of the Pathways Project. Personality and Mental Health; 2012;**6**(2):87–96.

Index